Vital Core Training

Improve Strength and Reduce Pain With Functional Movement

Leslee Bender

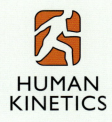

Library of Congress Cataloging-in-Publication Data

Names: Bender, Leslee author.
Title: Vital core training : improve strength and reduce pain with functional movement / Leslee Bender, ACSM, NASM, FAFS, PMA, BA.
Description: Champaign, IL : Human Kinetics, [2025] | Includes bibliographical references.
Identifiers: LCCN 2024003396 (print) | LCCN 2024003397 (ebook) | ISBN 9781718223745 (print ; alk. paper) | ISBN 9781718223752 (epub) | ISBN 9781718223769 (pdf)
Subjects: LCSH: Physical education and training. | Physical fitness. | Exercise. | Stretching exercises. | Muscle strength.
Classification: LCC GV341 .B424 2025 (print) | LCC GV341 (ebook) | DDC 796.071--dc23/eng/20240429
LC record available at https://lccn.loc.gov/2024003396
LC ebook record available at https://lccn.loc.gov/2024003397

ISBN: 978-1-7182-2374-5 (print)

Copyright © 2025 by Leslee Bender

Human Kinetics supports copyright. Copyright fuels scientific and artistic endeavor, encourages authors to create new works, and promotes free speech. Thank you for buying an authorized edition of this work and for complying with copyright laws by not reproducing, scanning, or distributing any part of it in any form without written permission from the publisher. You are supporting authors and allowing Human Kinetics to continue to publish works that increase the knowledge, enhance the performance, and improve the lives of people all over the world.

To report suspected copyright infringement of content published by Human Kinetics, contact us at **permissions@hkusa.com**. To request permission to legally reuse content published by Human Kinetics, please refer to the information at **https://US.HumanKinetics.com/pages/permissions-translations-faqs**.

This publication is written and published to provide accurate and authoritative information relevant to the subject matter presented. It is published and sold with the understanding that the author and publisher are not engaged in rendering legal, medical, or other professional services by reason of their authorship or publication of this work. If medical or other expert assistance is required, the services of a competent professional person should be sought.

The web addresses cited in this text were current as of February 2024, unless otherwise noted.

Senior Acquisitions Editor: Michelle Earle; **Developmental Editor:** Anne Hall; **Managing Editor:** Hannah Werner; **Copyeditor:** Heather Gauen Hutches; **Permissions Manager:** Laurel Mitchell; **Graphic Designer:** Dawn Sills; **Cover Designer:** Keri Evans; **Cover Design Specialist:** Susan Rothermel Allen; **Photographs (cover and interior):** © Human Kinetics; **Photo Production Specialist:** Amy M. Rose; **Photo Production Manager:** Jason Allen; **Senior Art Manager:** Kelly Hendren; **Illustrations:** © Human Kinetics; **Printer:** Versa Press

Human Kinetics books are available at special discounts for bulk purchase. Special editions or book excerpts can also be created to specification. For details, contact the Special Sales Manager at Human Kinetics.

Printed in the United States of America   10 9 8 7 6 5 4 3 2

The paper in this book is certified under a sustainable forestry program.

Human Kinetics	*United States and International*	*Canada*
1607 N. Market Street	Website: **US.HumanKinetics.com**	Website: **Canada.HumanKinetics.com**
Champaign, IL 61820	Email: info@hkusa.com	Email: info@hkcanada.com
USA	Phone: 1-800-747-4457	

E9227

Vital Core Training

Improve Strength and Reduce Pain With Functional Movement

Contents

Exercise Finder   vi
Foreword by Keli Roberts   ix
Acknowledgments   xi
Introduction   xii

PART I Foundations

CHAPTER 1
A New Functional Approach   3

Understand how small ball training provides spinal stability and increases mobility for all bodies.

CHAPTER 2
Core Essentials   9

Learn how the core muscles and fasciae function and move within the planes of motion.

PART II Exercises

CHAPTER 3
Vertical Exercises   23

Use gravity and the planes of motion to enhance body awareness through movement.

CHAPTER 4
Kneeling Exercises   59

Improve balance while using the ball to engage the core.

CHAPTER 5
Prone Exercises   79

Amplify hip and spine alignment with prone exercises.

CHAPTER 6
Side-Lying Exercises   93

Challenge the core and emphasize the obliques with side movements.

CHAPTER 7
Seated and Supine Exercises 113
Correct poor posture with exercises that support and strengthen the lower core muscles.

CHAPTER 8
Stretches 145
Learn to relax, boost mobility, and augment suppleness through stretching.

PART III Workouts

CHAPTER 9
Create Workouts 175
Learn how to combine exercises to create three levels of core essential workouts.

CHAPTER 10
Workouts for Better Posture and a Healthy Back 195
Follow sample workouts that address alignment dysfunctions and build core functionality.

CHAPTER 11
Core Workouts for Rotational Sports 219
Follow three sample workouts to complement popular recreational activities.

References   231
About the Author   233
Earn Continuing Education Credits/Units   234

Exercise Finder

Chapter 3

Anterior Hip Lengthening	28
Back Press to Wall	48
Back Press to Wall With Rotation	49
Balance (Ball Inside Knee)	54
Balance (Ball Outside Knee)	56
Balance (Ball Under Foot)	52
Calf and Posterior Hip Lengthening	27
Curtsy Lunge With Glider Disc	34
Hip Flexion and Balance	42
Lateral Flexion Against the Wall	50
Lunge	36
Lunge With Glider Disc	38
One-Handed Wall Press	46
Parallel Squat (Ball Between Hands)	30
Parallel Squat (Ball Between Thighs)	26
Squat to Balance	40
Squat With Lateral Flexion and Rotation	32
Staggered Squat (Ball Between Thighs)	29
Two-Handed Wall Press	44

Chapter 4

Hands and Knees (Ball Under Hand)	68
Hands and Knees (Ball Under Knees)	76
Hands and Knees With Glider Disc (Ball Between Thighs)	73
Hands and Knees With Hip Extension (Ball Under Hand)	70
Hands and Knees With Hip Extension (Ball Under Knee)	72
Hands and Knees With Hip Mobility With Glider Disc (Ball Between Thighs)	74
Hands and Knees With Toe Lifts (Ball Between Thighs)	75
Kneeling (Ball Between Thighs)	61
Kneeling With Knee Lifts (Ball Between Knees)	66

Kneeling With Lateral Flexion (Ball Between Thighs)	62
Kneeling With Rotation (Ball Between Thighs)	64

Chapter 5

Forearm Plank (Ball Between Hands)	90
Forearm Plank (Ball Under Chest)	81
Forearm Plank With Hip Extension (Ball Under Chest)	82
Forearm Plank With Hip Rotation With Glider Disc (Ball Between Thighs)	89
Plank (Ball Between Thighs)	83
Plank to Pike With Glider Disc (Ball Between Thighs)	88
Plank With Hip Extension (Ball Between Thighs)	84
Plank With Rotation (Ball Between Thighs)	86
Prone Hip Extension (Ball Between Ankles)	92
Prone Spinal Extension (Ball Under Hands)	91

Chapter 6

Forearm Side Plank (Ball Between Thighs)	100
One-Handed Side Plank (Ball Between Thighs)	102
Side-Lying Hip Abduction (Ball Under Head)	104
Side-Lying Hip Abduction (Ball Under Side)	106
Side-Lying Hip Abduction and Lateral Flexion (Ball Under Side)	108
Side-Lying Hip Abduction and Lateral Flexion With Glider Disc (Ball Under Side)	110
Side-Lying Hip Adduction (Ball Between Ankles)	98
Side-Lying Lateral Flexion (Ball Under Side)	94
Side-Lying Lateral Flexion With Glider Disc (Ball Under Side)	96

Chapter 7

Bridge (Ball Between Knees)	128
Bridge (Ball on Thighs)	132
Bridge (Ball Under Foot)	130
Bridge (Ball Under Sacrum)	127
Bridge With Hip Flexion (Ball on Thigh)	134
Hip and Knee Extension (Ball Under Sacrum)	138
Hip Flexion (Ball on Thigh)	140

Chapter 7 *(continued)*

Hip Flexion With Toe Taps (Ball on Thighs)	142
Seated Anterior and Lateral Core Lengthening (Ball Behind Mid Back)	126
Seated Anterior and Lateral Core Rotation (Ball Behind Low Back)	122
Seated Anterior and Lateral Core Rotation With Glider Disc (Ball Behind Low Back)	124
Seated Anterior Core Lengthening (Ball Behind Low Back)	116
Seated Anterior Core Lengthening (Ball Behind Mid Back)	115
Seated Anterior Core Lengthening With Chair	118
Seated Anterior Core Lengthening With Glider Disc (Ball Behind Low Back)	120
Toe Taps (Ball Under Sacrum)	136

Chapter 8

Butterfly Stretch	164
Hamstring Stretch	168
Hip Flexor Stretch	166
Inner Thigh Stretch	154
Pectoralis Stretch	159
Posterior Cross Lunge	152
Side Bend	148
Side Bend With Legs Crossed	150
Side-Lying Stretch	160
Supine Rotation	162
Thread the Needle	158
Upper Back and Chest Stretch	170
Vertical Rotation	156

Chapter 9

Breath Work	178
Dynamic Stretches	180

Foreword

I had the pleasure of first meeting Leslee Bender at the 2004 IDEA International Convention, where we were both presenting. It was at that time that I realized just how like-minded we were; we both focused on safe and effective training for all populations and all needs. We share a no-nonsense approach, with a philosophy of teaching movements that matter and with functional exercises that enhance posture, alignment, and strength and decrease pain and injury risk.

In 2007, I attended Leslee's Bender Ball certification in Reno, and that's when I discovered how to train effectively with a small ball. It was clear from that moment that the depth of her knowledge and skill in practical application were profound. I wish I had this book way back then! It would have been the perfect addition to reinforce what I learned from that valuable course.

I am still amazed by the versatility and effectiveness of small ball training! It's simple to incorporate small ball training into my group fitness classes and include them in my one-on-one sessions with many of my clients. I'm sure it will be the same for you with the exercises in this in-depth book!

In my personal training business, I work with a wide variety of clients, most with special needs due to health complications and age-related issues. For clients with Parkinson's disease, multiple sclerosis (MS), hip and knee replacements, heart disease, osteoporosis, and lower back and neck pain as well as for cancer survivors, I have found the small ball to be an essential tool for training postural issues, alignment, and more.

This book incorporates many of the moves I learned in that 2007 certification. I've found this functional approach to movement to be effective for a wide variety of clients, no matter what gender, fitness level, or ability. In fact, my client with MS benefited enormously in strengthening her core and balance with many of Leslee's exercises. Additionally, I found the small ball to be an excellent tool for my client with osteoporosis because I could protect her fragile spine and still effectively strengthen her core.

On a personal note, in 2014, my left shoulder was replaced due to a cycling accident. The recovery was long and slow, and for many months, conventional core training, such as planks and side planks, was not possible. I was able to incorporate many small ball movements to maintain and build my core strength. This experience enabled me to help many individuals struggling with shoulder injuries to find effective methods to train the core without involving the shoulder girdle.

In this book, you will find a huge collection of small ball training exercises organized into logical categories. Just like I learned in the certification so many years ago, these timeless, effective, and safe exercises are appropriate for multiple populations to achieve their diverse goals. With clearly explained, intelligent cueing, Leslee makes these moves accessible and doable. In addition to gaining access to a massive movement library, you'll also enhance your ability to coach and communicate effectively!

This valuable book provides not only great exercises but also easy-to-follow, goal-specific programs that will make a difference beyond aesthetics. In my more than 37 years of teaching and training, I have seen that form follows function. Leslee's functional approach to training builds a body that moves and feels better! You'll learn to enhance alignment and posture so that it's possible to decrease pain and injury risk. And when you move better and feel better, you look better!

Keli Roberts, ACSM-EP, ACE CPT, GFI, HC, NASM CES
2003 IDEA International Instructor of the Year
2007 National Fitness Hall of Fame Inductee

Acknowledgments

I would like to thank all of those in the industry with whom I have worked and had such great opportunities to train. As a graduate of the Gray Institute of Applied Functional Science, I continue to dedicate my admiration to them for their method of training the body authentically. I am also grateful for Savvier Fitness, who made it possible for the Bender Method to be named the 2006 Infomercial of the Year, and for IDEA Health and Fitness, who recognized me as the 2020 Personal Trainer of the Year. And finally, I am grateful for all of the clients with whom I have worked.

Introduction

Welcome! In this book, you will enhance your journey as a trainer by learning how to use a small ball in exercises that strengthen the core while protecting the back. As trainers, we need to diversify our knowledge to include modalities of training that are effective and functional for all bodies. The focus on high-intensity training programs is now shifting toward a mind–body approach based on systematic applications for the body. This program embraces this approach with a functional method that can be practiced by all movement specialists. No matter the age, gender, or ability level of our clients, we have the choice to train with a purpose that leads to greater success.

Leslee's Journey

I have been in the industry for over four decades and have several credentials (ACSM; NASM; FAFS; FAI; NPCP; ACE; BA; UNR; RealRyder; YogaFit 1, 2, and 3; Polestar Pilates), and I believe that knowledge is power and education is the key. As the creator of the Bender Method of core training, I was the first to introduce a small fitness ball to the field at a time when the large Swiss ball was booming in the market. I have traveled the world observing many ways of delivering fitness programs and discovered that most students want to live an active, happy life.

I began my career when the 1980s craze of high-impact aerobics was the primary modality of fitness. Sadly, I was one of many trainers who for years taught primarily high-intensity and step classes, with a blend of terrible core training, unaware of the damage I was doing to not only my own body but those of the clients who participated in my classes. We did not yet know about or understand the importance of functional training such as foam rolling and flexibility training—we could have saved millions of knees, hips, and backs had we known. As a recipient of a total knee replacement in 2019, I fully understand how, had I trained differently, my surgery likely could have been avoided. Now, as we look at the future of fitness and wellness, there is better research on how to train for longevity. The vast majority of my clients are now interested in active aging, and I have come to realize that my knee replacement has made me a more empathetic trainer. A joint replacement is not easy to recover from, and preventive training is certainly more desirable. It is now my deepest desire to help my clients protect their backs and strengthen their cores so that they will live functional, pain-free lives.

Scope and Content of This Book

This book will change the way you train yourself and your clients for a functional life. Unlike many other programs that simply teach how to do exercises, the content I share here helps movement specialists understand why and how the body responds to different types of training strategies using a small ball. You will learn how to combine myofascial lengthening techniques with intelligent movement and empowering language to enhance stability, mobility, flexibility, balance, body awareness, strength, endurance, self-esteem, and confidence.

As you read this book, you will do the following:

- Experience an innovative training method to feel your body move authentically using myofascial lengthening and release techniques in combination with challenging functional exercises
- Expand your skills and techniques as you learn an easy-to-implement core movement training system that delivers profound results for people of all ages and abilities
- Decrease pain through integrated techniques
- Develop a deeper understanding of the connection between the breath and the muscles as they relate to many types of movement
- Learn to coach participants to truly feel their body move using language that builds body awareness, self-esteem, and confidence
- Understand the science and research to appreciate the rationale behind the core training system
- Select exercises that train movement based on the planes of motion to create a body that moves with freedom and flow
- Be able to evaluate the needs and abilities of all clients
- Create classes based around client goals and individual learning styles
- Devise cues that support different types of learners (visual, auditory, and kinesthetic)
- Improve your critical thinking skills

As I have grown in my education and experience as a fitness professional, it is my desire that we begin to truly look at individual needs, body types, and goals with a critical eye. Too many programs are based on aesthetics instead of the health and functionality of the client; even today, there are too many injuries that could be avoided. We are in a new world of the Internet, where the unsuspecting client may watch unsafe programming and exercises delivered by an uncertified individual. This is where we come in, as educated professionals delivering programming that is truly safe and effective for all levels of clients who desire a strong core and a pain-free body. I am excited for you to embark on this journey to expand your awareness of the human body and how to move efficiently, safely, and with intention.

/ PART I

Foundations

CHAPTER 1

A New Functional Approach

The concepts in this book represent a new approach to training the core by applying a functional method for all participants, resulting in less pain and better strength and mobility. There are many core training programs that are based primarily on aesthetics rather than function, but when we consider the age, abilities, and goals of individual clients, we can choose the appropriate exercises that will truly enhance their lives. Here you will learn how and why using a small ball with functional exercises protects the back, increases core activation in both the deep and superficial muscles, and lengthens the fasciae for mobility and stability.

Benefits of Learning the Methods of Vital Core Training

With the methods you will learn in this book, you will achieve better body awareness, more core strength, less pain, and a more functional approach to training. Your body will adapt to the techniques and respond accordingly, resulting in healthier behaviors and an improved quality of life.

Physical and Physiological Benefits

The physical benefits of an exercise program can vary dramatically depending on the nature of the training. For example, the body adapts differently to running than walking because the impact on the joints is harsher. When we train in a modality that is safe on our joints and does not create pain, we can move more easily. The core exercises in this book are designed to benefit the body's natural alignment so all the parts of the body can do their jobs successfully.

Many people have a tendency to not consider how one part of the body affects others. For example, being in spinal flexion for long periods of time puts stress on the back, which affects the entire body. If someone sits at a desk all day, then does poor core training such as supine crunches, the physiological body adapts to being in a flexed position. In turn, the back starts to hurt and it becomes harder to get oxygen into the cells as a result of not sitting correctly. In essence, the body adapts to the sitting more than to the core training. By placing the small ball behind the low back, extension is created, resulting in 408 percent greater core activation than supine crunches alone (Petrofsky et al. 2007).

If we can view how the body works synergistically, then we can create change. One of the hardest concepts for individuals to realize is that overtraining the physiological body decreases immunity and leads to exhaustion, muscle soreness, and eventually injuries. And once an injury occurs, it can take a long time to recover. Therefore, cross-training, mind–body work, functional training, and, above all, rest will allow the body to function at its optimum level of efficiency.

Behavioral Benefits

If a program is too difficult and painful, it is not uncommon for a client to become discouraged and quit. When a client starts a program that is functionally challenging and safe for their body and abilities, they will likely start to see results and stick with it. Results are individual and will vary depending on following the program, but when a program is designed for success for all individuals, the potential for a positive outcome is greater.

This program is designed with regressions and progressions for all levels of clients, allowing individuals to progress at their own pace. Using a small ball for all exercises also provides enough of a challenge that even the strongest core junkie will feel accomplished and successful.

Why the Small Ball?

The mini stability ball, or small ball, was designed to protect the low back when used correctly during exercise, allowing the body to lengthen rather than shorten. It can be used with clients of all levels, abilities, genders, and ages to provide stability for the lumbar spine and mobility for the thoracic spine. It also helps maintain alignment of the knees, provides kinesthetic feedback, and serves as a visual tool.

Incorporating the small ball into the functional training you teach to clients will allow them to train more efficiently and with less risk of injury. For example, abdominal crunches have traditionally been used to train the core muscles of the body. However, these supine crunches compress the spine and provide only low levels of muscle activity. Performing exercises with a small ball behind the back increases stability, mobility, and core activation, allowing for greater extension and increased muscle work.

Don't just take my word for it that using a small ball is effective! Research comparing core muscle activity during exercise using a mini stability ball (small ball), abdominal crunches on the floor, and abdominal crunches on a Swiss ball also found the small ball had effective results (Petrofsky et al. 2007). In this study, three levels of core exercise were tested with the mini stability ball. The results showed that crunches on the Swiss ball used approximately 50 percent more muscle recruitment per second of exercise than the floor crunches. The lightest exercise with the mini stability ball (sitting crunches with the ball behind the back) was about equal to half of the work per second as floor crunches. However, the most intense exercises with the mini stability ball equaled as much as four times the work per second as abdominal crunches. The greatest difference in the mini stability ball exercise was seen when the degree of flexion and extension was increased from 50 to 90 degrees. This degree of flexion cannot be accomplished with standard floor crunches or with the Swiss ball, thereby giving the mini stability ball a significant advantage in working the muscles harder and at a better range of motion.

Ultimately, this study demonstrated how much more efficient using a small ball for core work can be. The more accustomed your clients are to correctly performing these movements in training, the more natural the movements become, making it more likely that they will move more efficiently in their daily lives as well.

Conscious and Subconscious Understanding

When the body adapts to performing a task, it becomes a habit. We all have subconscious movement patterns. Over time, faulty movement patterns (such as sitting at a computer with poor posture) can lead to dysfunction and injuries. However, once a faulty movement pattern is detected, then conscious changes can be made. When a task is performed routinely, it becomes subconscious. For example, when a squat has been practiced correctly over and over, the subconscious mind directs the body to also pick up an object from the floor correctly. This is a positive shift for any client looking to improve overall well-being.

The more programming mimics everyday activities, the better the outcome. Many exercises do not translate to function, but rather are based on aesthetics or fads. For example, tucking the pelvis and tightening the glutes completely restricts all movements of the hip, which does not translate to daily activities such as squatting and lifting. Remember that the body adapts to consistent training, whether functional or dysfunctional. Therefore, exercise prescriptions and specific cues for success should be well thought out for each client. When you take a client through functional movements, you help them create healthy movement patterns that will improve their ability to live functionally and without pain.

The Types of Learners

Using a client's preferred method of learning allows us to ensure that they can understand and perform an exercise task to the best of their ability. Making sure to use visual, kinesthetic, and auditory cues will provide this necessary feedback to the client.

Kinesthetic

A kinesthetic learner needs hands-on attention and correction to ensure the proper alignment. They may be slower to execute a movement correctly, but the use of a small ball will help greatly. For example, placing the small ball behind the lower back while sitting immediately reminds them to align their posture. When this individual trains regularly in correct alignment, the body adapts to better posture, which results in greater functionality.

Auditory

An auditory learner needs very clear and concise instructions to perform a task—the more precise, the better. It is imperative to guide them on the correct setup. Cues such as "engage your glutes" rather than "squeeze your booty" can be effective to help perform the movement in correct alignment. Explain where and how to feel the exercise and let them process the cue for a moment.

Visual

A visual learner needs to see how a movement is performed and then can mimic it to the best of their ability. As a trainer, you should only demonstrate a few times, not consider this time for your own workout—too often trainers are looking at themselves and not observing their clients. The visual learner most likely has good body awareness and does not need to watch a trainer do a movement over and over. Once they have demonstrated, the trainer can work on other cues.

Success as a Trainer

Have you ever been in a class where you were looking at the clock, wishing it would end faster? On the other hand, have you ever taken a class that you wished would never end? We have all probably experienced both of these scenarios as students or clients ourselves. To create the latter experience, a great trainer should keep good energy in the room, look at their clients for feedback, and be present without exception. If a trainer is not paying attention and clients are struggling, injuries can occur.

The following best practices can help you deliver world-class experiences each time you work with clients.

- Remember that you are not there to perform; this is not your workout.
- Understand the purpose of each movement.
- Always face your clients. Look at each individual and the way they execute movements.
- Coach, cue, and connect with each client.
- Use specific, descriptive language when coaching clients.
- Teach both the *how* and the *why*.
- Be positive.
- Compliment clients' success.
- Know when to refer a client to a medical professional.
- Never put a client in danger with a contraindicated exercise.

Professional verbiage is the language used intelligently to coach, cue, connect, and compliment a client. It's essential for helping clients find success. Table 1.1 shows examples of preferred phrases for teaching someone how to get the most out of each movement.

TABLE 1.1 Intelligent Cuing

Intelligent cuing with meaning	Overused language
"Engage your glutes"	"Squeeze your booty"
"Experience what you are feeling in the front of the body"	"Tighten your core till it burns"
"Feel your body move authentically"	"Feel the burn"
"Lengthen your body"; "Feel your body lengthen"	"Tighten your body up"
"Explore the movement"	"Push, push, push"
"Do what feels good"	"Go for the burn"
"Work within your range"	"Go harder"

The Breath

Breathing is a necessity of life. When you inhale, oxygen is carried to the blood cells. When you exhale, carbon dioxide is released as waste. Improper breathing can upset this exchange of oxygen and carbon dioxide and contribute to anxiety, panic attacks, fatigue, and other physical and emotional disturbances.

The diaphragm is a dome-shaped muscle that separates the chest from the stomach and facilitates breathing (figure 1.1). It contracts and flattens with inhalation, creating a vacuum that draws air into the lungs, and relaxes and rises with exhalation, pushing air out of the lungs.

When executing an exercise, inhale through the nose to prepare and exhale through the mouth on the exertion. Encourage clients to breathe normally, inhaling to prepare and practicing a slight exhalation during exertion. However, they should not force it. Too often, clients become overwhelmed with paying attention to the breath and compromise the actual movement. Model a subtle and effortless breath.

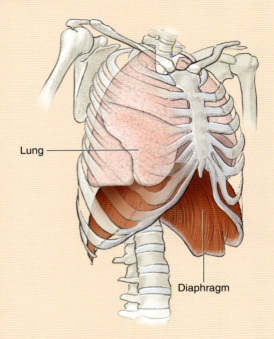

FIGURE 1.1 The diaphragm.

Vital core training using a small ball provides physical and physiological benefits—such as less pain and better strength and mobility while protecting the low back from injury—as well as behavioral benefits. When a client starts to feel the correct way of performing an exercise, it can translate to other activities, such as squatting down and even breathing correctly. And when exercise and everyday tasks are done successfully, this can lead to a dramatically more positive attitude in life. With repeated training, conscious movement becomes subconscious and good habits are built.

Clients can find success through kinesthetic, auditory, or visual feedback provided by trainers during exercise. As a trainer, knowing how your students learn is vital for success and progression. Trainers must also know the why behind each exercise they include in the client's programming and should use intelligent cues with clients. Too often, trainers use ineffective language, which can lead to either pain or injuries.

CHAPTER 2

Core Essentials

The abdominal or core muscles are unique. The core is involved in all movements from vertical to supine and should be thought of as the body's support system. Whether someone is picking something up or doing an exercise, the entire kinetic chain is engaged as an integrated system. When all these moving parts work in harmony, we can live more functional, pain-free lives and engage in activities such as gardening or sports that make life more fulfilling.

Because the core muscles, in particular the abdominal muscles, are used to stabilize the spine, they are correlated to the incidence of back injury. When core muscles are weak, even simple tasks such as bending over can incur an injury (McGill 2002). Strengthening these muscles therefore not only has strong central effects in the body, such as improved cardiovascular functioning, but also reduces the risk of injury by increasing back stability. This is important because back injuries are a major cause of dysfunction and pain and cost the American public billions of dollars each year in medical care (Julia 2023). These injuries can first occur early in life and, if not recognized or treated, can reoccur frequently.

The abdominal muscles have several important jobs in addition to stabilization, including the following:

- Helping with essential bodily functions, including urinating, coughing, and sneezing
- Increasing intra-abdominal pressure to facilitate childbirth
- Supporting and protecting internal organs

Unilateral Exercise Benefits

We all have a dominant or stronger side of the body; therefore, it is good to focus on strengthening the weaker side as a way to increase symmetry. Unilateral exercises—those that are performed on one side of the body at a time—can be useful to help clients identify and strengthen these weaker areas. Creating better balance can reduce the risk of injuries and improve performance. Many of the exercises in this book will help increase symmetry and achieve balance.

The Abdominal Muscles

There are five main muscles in the abdomen: The two vertical muscles, rectus abdominis and pyramidalis (located under the rectus abdominis), are located toward the middle of the body, and the three flat muscles, the external obliques, internal obliques, and transversus abdominis, are stacked on top of each other and situated toward the sides of the trunk (figure 2.1).

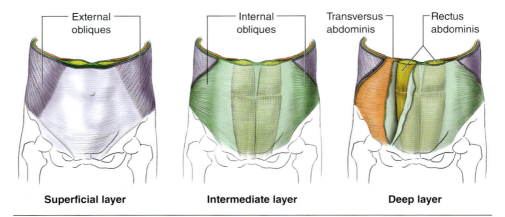

FIGURE 2.1 The primary abdominal muscles.

Pyramidalis

This vertical muscle is small and shaped like a triangle. It's located very low in the pelvis under the rectus abdominis and helps maintain internal abdominal pressure. The pyramidalis is frequently thought of as the lower abs, but in actuality, the pyramidalis and the rectus abdominis work in conjunction and cannot be isolated when training.

Rectus Abdominis

This pair of muscles goes down the middle of the abdomen from the ribs to the front of the pelvis and may form what looks like a "six-pack" when someone has a lean body. They hold the internal organs in place and provide stability during all body movements. These muscles flex the spine when supine and decelerate extension when leaning back. When the small ball is placed behind the back, the rectus abdominis muscles provide extension rather than just flexion against gravity.

External Obliques

The external obliques are a pair of large, flat muscles, one on each side of the rectus abdominis. They run from the lower half of the ribs around and down to the pelvis. They are the outermost of the three types of flat muscles and cover the internal obliques and the anterior ribs. The external obliques allow the trunk to rotate and extend.

Internal Obliques

The internal obliques are a pair of muscles on top of the external obliques, just inside the hip bones. Like the external obliques, they are located on the sides of the rectus abdominis, running from the sides of the trunk toward the middle. They work with the external oblique muscles to allow the trunk to rotate.

Transversus Abdominis

Located near the spinal column and deeper than the other muscles, the transversus abdominis muscle wraps around the lower part of the torso and is known as the body's corset. It influences respiration but does not create movement such as flexion or extension. During muscle contraction, the fibers are pulled toward the center of the body, tightening the pelvic floor and organs toward one another and creating balance relative to the core. Training the core correctly increases muscle strength, which, combined with good posture and alignment, will improve posture and help relieve pressure on the spine, which may, in turn, lead to less pain.

The Back Muscles

The posterior core muscles are a group of muscles located in the back of the body (figure 2.2). They include the multifidus, quadratus lumborum, and erector spinae muscles. These muscles play a crucial role in maintaining posture, stabilizing the spine, and facilitating movement, including extension and lateral flexion. The posterior muscles also work synergistically with the anterior core of the body to ensure neutral spine, described next.

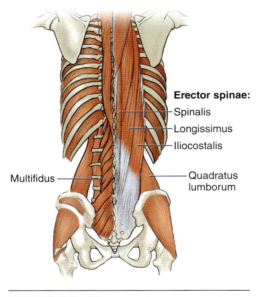

FIGURE 2.2 The posterior core muscles.

Defining Neutral Spine

What does *neutral spine* mean, and why is it so important? The definition is quite simple: Neutral spine is good posture—the position in which the back and neck are placed under the least amount of stress and strain, allowing them to function properly and without damage or pain (figure 2.3). This is also the position of the spine in which the least amount of effort is necessary. Think about young children: They run and play effortlessly and without pain. However, as we age, habitual postures, stress, injuries, lifestyle, and ineffective workouts will influence spine health and cause issues if not addressed.

You may have been taught to cue clients in your fitness classes to pull in their abs or tuck the pelvis. These cues are incorrect—and useless if you're trying to develop a well-functioning body. All exercises in this program are based on neutral spine and do not involve tucking the pelvis, which restricts

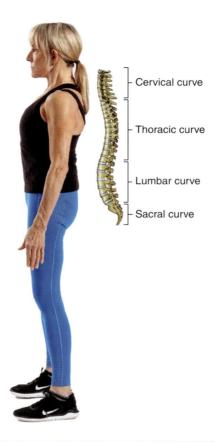

FIGURE 2.3 An example of a neutral spine and the parts of the spine. Good posture features a natural convex (outward) curve in the thoracic vertebrae and sacrum, and a concave (inward) curve in the cervical and lumbar vertebrae.

movement and can cause back pain. The body was meant to move authentically. When in neutral spine, movement becomes easier to accomplish with less strain on the rest of the body's joints.

Postural Issues

Postural issues can be greatly corrected given the appropriate exercise and equipment. There are many causes of poor posture, many of which people are not even aware of. The unsuspecting client may perform exercises that have actually negatively contributed to their poor posture or even led to injuries. This is where you as a trainer can make a big difference! When a trainer assesses an individual's posture, they can be a great influence on proper alignment.

This book includes exercises that can directly correlate to improved posture and decreased pain.

Poor posture can be caused by a number of factors, including the following:

- Poor ergonomics when seated
- Weight gain and inactivity
- Lack of awareness of bad posture
- Use of technology that puts the body in a compromised position
- Performing exercises that contribute to postural deficiencies
- Hereditary conditions such as scoliosis

The two most common types of poor posture are kyphosis and lordosis (figure 2.4).

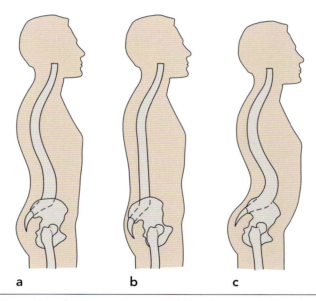

FIGURE 2.4 Examples of *(a)* normal posture, *(b)* kyphosis, and *(c)* lordosis.

Kyphosis

Kyphosis is a pronounced outward curve of the upper back and an anterior head carriage (i.e., slouching). This position places stress on the cervical spine. It can sometimes be the result of overtraining the chest or carrying more weight in the abdominal area. Kyphosis can be characterized by the following:

- Forward head carriage
- Tight pectoralis and deltoids
- Tight glutes

- Tight hamstrings
- Supinated feet
- Weak postural muscles

Common causes of kyphosis include the following:

- Training that includes too much flexion
- Not enough flexibility training
- Insufficient lengthening of the anterior chain

Avoiding supine crunches is advised for an individual with kyphosis because they cause more flexion of the spine. Using the small ball will allow for extension and rotation in certain exercises that cannot be achieved by simply lying on the floor. This can help improve general flexibility and that of the thoracic spine, as well as promote better posture when used in seated exercises.

Lordosis

Lordosis is an exaggerated inward curve of the spine, or swayback, that can lead to excess pressure on the spine. If left untreated or ignored, it can cause back pain, especially later in life. This posture is more common in women because of the shape of the pelvis. Lordosis is characterized by the following:

- Anterior carriage of the pelvis
- Anterior carriage of the hips
- Tight hip flexors
- Tight calves
- Weak anterior core
- Weak glutes
- Weak hamstrings
- Pronated feet
- Valgus knees

Common causes of lordosis include the following:

- Training that involves excessive flexion of the spine and overutilizes the hip flexors (such as crunches or any other supine exercise)
- Wearing high heels
- Pronated feet
- Pregnancy

The correct core exercise program can help alleviate the effects of lordosis. The small ball can be used in all seated exercises, in vertical exercises such as squats to align the knees, and in specific stretches to lengthen the hip flexors.

It can also be used in certain core exercises to help disengage the hip flexors and allow the anterior core to work more efficiently. Because sitting for long periods shortens the hip flexors, even simply getting up and stretching will provide benefits.

The Role of Fascia in Posture and Movement

The fascia are among the body's most crucial components for mobility, stability, agility, balance, and resilience, yet they are often completely overlooked in fitness. Fascia are made up of layers of connective tissue beneath the skin, with liquid between each layer called *hyaluronan* (figure 2.5). These tissues attach, stabilize, strengthen, maintain blood vessel integrity, separate muscles, and enclose different organs. In addition to providing internal structure, fasciae have nerves that make them sensitive.

Fascia is designed to stretch and lengthen with movement. However, it can thicken and become sticky as a result of lack of movement and sitting too much. When fascia becomes dehydrated and tightens around muscles, this can decrease mobility and create pain. Utilizing the small ball in many exercises will help lengthen this tissue. Motion is lotion is a great way to look at it!

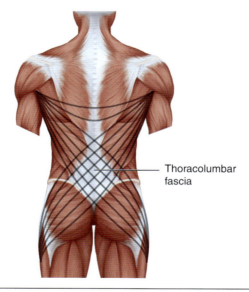

FIGURE 2.5 An example of how fascia is layered with muscle tissue, in this case the posterior muscles of the back and upper legs. The relationship between fascia and muscle creates structural tension that allows for the body to move with stability and mobility.

Keeping your fascia healthy has many benefits. You'll move more easily, have better range of motion, and experience less pain. Here are ways to promote healthy fascia.

- *Move constantly.* In addition to a consistent core routine, it's important to be active throughout the day. Placing the ball behind the back while sitting improves posture and allows you to do extension movement, which helps fascia stay supple. Getting up and performing vertical core movements keeps the body energized as well.
- *Stretch and lengthen.* Stretching is essential to good health. It reduces the risk of inflammation and structural problems in the body. In part II of this book, you will be introduced to many exercises that promote lengthening the tissue.
- *Pay attention to posture.* Slumping over a desk or a phone or walking awkwardly to compensate for an injury can cause fascia to tighten. When sitting for long periods of time, think of your fascia and muscles shortening to compensate for the gravity placed on the spine. If you then do crunches for core training, you have to shorten the muscles to flex the spine—and without the ball behind the back there is no extension, further contributing to shortened muscles and a dysfunctional body. Although this is common, you can train the core muscles in a way that improves posture and reduces the risk of dysfunction. Posture leads to vitality when you move authentically.

Fascia and Proprioception

Fascia may also play a role in proprioception, or the body's ability to sense movement and body position. Sensory receptors called *proprioceptors*, found chiefly in muscles, tendons, joints, and fascia, detect motion or the position of the body or a limb by responding to stimuli such as gravity and ground reaction. For example, lengthening movements during propulsion such as walking or running stimulate the proprioceptors to decelerate the body without conscious effort.

Proprioceptors play an important role in developing good posture and efficient movement patterns. Specifically, movement and touch affect and stimulate the proprioceptors. When there is lack of movement, it affects their resilience. For example, when standing up after sitting for a long period, the body will feel stiff. When fascia are exposed to compression, injury, dehydration, overuse, and imbalanced motion, they become thick, inflamed, knotted, and twisted. The result is a lack of blood flow, lack of oxygen flow, decreased range of motion, and increased tension and pain. This causes loss of balance, body awareness, and mobility.

Planes of Motion

The planes of motion allow us to understand how the body reacts to gravity and loading in movement (figure 2.6). When you understand the planes of motion, you can then create exercises based on the needs of your clients.

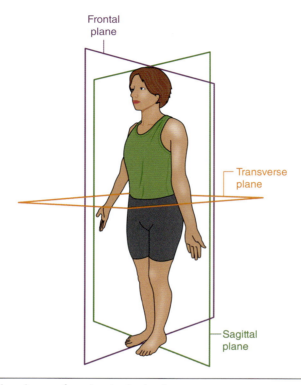

FIGURE 2.6 The planes of motion in the body.

Sagittal Plane

The sagittal plane divides the body into anterior (front) and posterior (back) halves. For example, when you hyperextend the spine, you are lengthening the anterior part of the body and shortening the posterior, just as when you flex forward you are lengthening the posterior part of the body and shortening the anterior. Unfortunately, many trainers focus too much on teaching crunches and excessive spinal flexion in a supine position, which shortens the anterior parts of the body and can affect the quality of the sagittal plane. Teaching effective exercises in this plane of motion is the perfect opportunity to lengthen the body.

Here are some examples of movements in the sagittal plane:

- Performing squats with the small ball between the knees
- Lunging anteriorly or posteriorly when reaching upward
- Lunging anteriorly or posteriorly when reaching below the knee
- Performing seated core work with the small ball

Frontal Plane

The frontal plane divides the body from right to left, as in lateral flexion or abduction and adduction. For example, when you flex the spine to the right, you are lengthening the left side of the body. When you abduct the right hip, you are lengthening the adductors. Using the ball allows the body to lengthen in core exercises, unlike a supine lateral crunch, which only shortens the side of body and causes misalignments from right to left. This plane of motion is affected by gravity as well, which can be used for oblique training.

Here are examples of movements in the frontal plane:

- Vertical lateral flexion
- Vertical abduction of the hip
- Vertical adduction of the hip
- Side plank using the small ball
- Side lateral flexion using the small ball

Transverse Plane

The transverse or axial plane divides the body into top and bottom halves. It is involved in rotational movement in the torso, shoulder, and hip. Unlike the other two planes of motion, transverse exercises are not influenced by gravity and require a conscious effort. When not combined with the other planes, moving in the transverse plane is when clients will most likely injure the lumbar spine with a quick twisting motion. It is vital to use the other planes of motion for function, which can be facilitated with the small ball.

Here are examples of movements in the transverse plane:

- Vertical rotation holding the small ball
- Internal and external rotation of the shoulder and hip

All the planes of motion are part of human movement. Training in all three planes is therefore necessary for daily activities from walking to gardening to playing a favorite sport. If you were to only train in one, then the muscles in that plane of motion would become stronger, but your movement would not be functional. Looking at the body as a whole rather than in parts when considering the ways in which the body moves will help you develop elasticity, functionality, and flexibility in all dimensions.

Knowing the important role of each of the core muscles is vital to success when training the body for decreased pain and increased strength, mobility, and stability. For example, performing endless crunches would only lead to shortening the rectus abdominis and compromising posture, while training the core intelligently leads to better alignment, mobility, and stability. When training, considering postural issues is critical. Understanding the role fascia plays is equally important because healthy, elastic, and resilient fascia allows the body to move more freely and without pain or injury. The goal is lengthening the fascia, and this can be accomplished with the use of specific exercises, which should be chosen based on a thorough understanding of the planes of motion.

PART II

Exercises

CHAPTER 3

Vertical Exercises

In this chapter you will learn how to train the core from the ground up, taking advantage of the planes of motion discussed in chapter 2. It is important to allow your clients to find their personal range of motion, one that does not create discomfort in the knees or hips. Using the ball for these core movements allows for variations, regressions, and progressions with improved core awareness.

When initiating any of the movements, it is important to keep a neutral spine and hinge from the hips to protect both the back and knees. Many of us have performed dysfunctional core exercises in the past, but this can be reversed through the use of proper techniques and purposeful movements. For example, supine crunches were once thought of as the main modality of activating the core at the end of a fitness class, and now we know that lying on the back does not translate to function in daily activities and that flexion for long periods of time is not good for the spine or posture. Creating a conscious movement allows the body to adapt to good alignment in other daily activities. Just as athletes constantly practice good techniques to be their best, we create muscle memory by practicing pain-free functional movements.

The exercises and stretches are color coded. Exercises in green are for all levels of participants. Exercises in blue are slightly more challenging yet appropriate for most participants. Exercises in red are for higher-level participants looking for a more challenging exercise.

You will find that most of the exercises in this text are suitable for everyone. However, if an exercise seems too difficult, then alignment or outcome can be compromised; therefore, make sure the exercise feels good to the client's body so the goal can be achieved. Keep in mind that good alignment and form are more important than anything else with all exercises in this program.

Benefits and Cues

Using the ball with vertical exercises provides several benefits. The small ball can

- help align the hips,
- activate the deep pelvic floor muscles,
- help gauge range of motion, and
- improve balance and provide kinesthetic feedback.

The following alignment cues should be reviewed before undertaking the exercises:

- Make sure to have good balance when standing before initiating any movement, whether barefoot or wearing shoes.
- Keep a neutral spine *(a)*.
- Do not tuck the pelvis or tighten the glutes *(b)*.
- Think of lengthening the body throughout the movements.
- Engage and align the body in all movements.
- Move within an appropriate range of motion *(c, d)*.

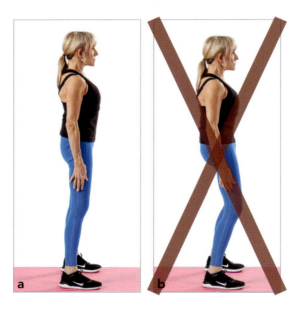

Vertical Exercises   25

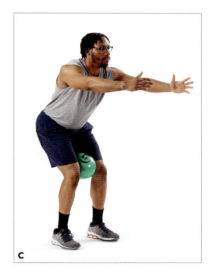
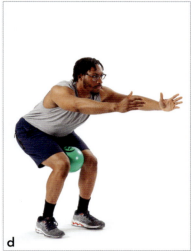

- Feel the movement as described.
- Move slowly and deliberately with the intention of achieving the desired outcome.
- Breathe to increase mobility in the core.
- Do not squeeze the ball so much that it creates dysfunctional posture *(e)*. Applying light pressure on the ball will maintain good alignment *(f)*.

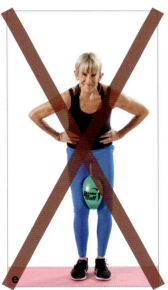
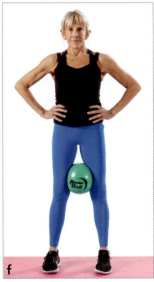

Parallel Squat (Ball Between Thighs)

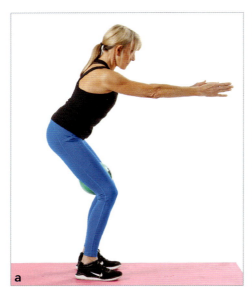 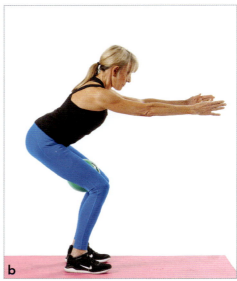

Benefits
Squatting with the ball allows the hips and knees to be aligned while activating the adductors and pelvic floor.

Instructions
1. Begin with the feet hip-width apart, the arms straight in front of the chest, and the ball held between the thighs about 4 inches (10 cm) above the knees.
2. Place the weight in the heels, hinge at the hips, and flex the knees as you lower into a squat, feeling the glutes lengthen.
3. Upon returning to standing, engage the inner thighs and pelvic floor as you stand.
4. Inhale to lower, causing the pelvic floor to drop; exhale to stand.
5. Perform 6 to 8 repetitions.

Alignment Cues
- Keep the spine lengthened and in neutral position.
- Do not tuck or tighten the glutes or arch the back.
- Imagine you are sitting in a chair as you lower into the squat.
- Keep your gaze forward.
- Keep your weight over the heels.
- As you return to a standing position, think of being tall.

Vertical Exercises   27

Calf and Posterior Hip Lengthening

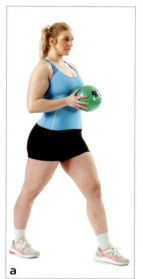
a

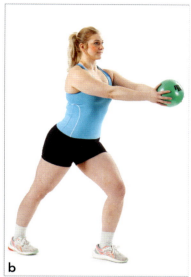
b

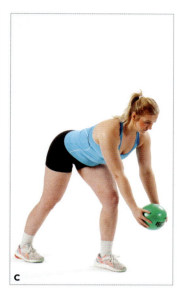
c

Benefits
Lengthening these specific areas of the body allows for better mobility and stability in the kinetic chain, and the ball provides a visual tool to keep you engaged in the movement.

Instructions
1. Begin with the feet hip-width apart. Hold the ball in both hands in front of the chest and inhale.
2. Step back approximately 2 feet (0.5 m) with the right foot, toes facing forward, exhaling to initiate the movement.
3. Extend the arms so the ball is in front of you and flex the left knee until the right calf engages and lengthens.
4. Keeping the arms straight, move the ball slightly below the left knee to feel the left glute and hamstring lengthen.
5. Move the arms to a position parallel to the shoulders, then lower the hands below the front knee before returning to the starting position.
6. Perform 6 to 8 repetitions on each side.

Alignment Cues
- Keep the spine lengthened and in neutral position.
- Stay within your range of motion.
- Keep the back heel on the ground and the feet parallel, toes facing forward.

Anterior Hip Lengthening

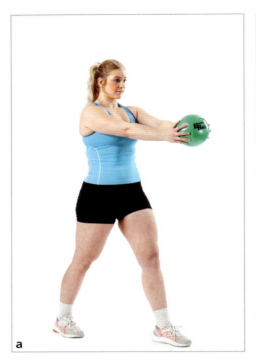 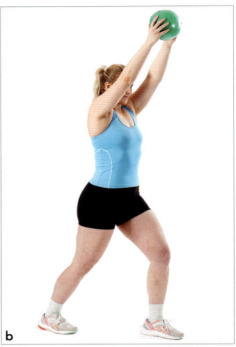

Benefits
Because the hips are often tight from sitting, it is helpful to lengthen the hip flexors prior to most exercises.

Instructions
1. Begin with the feet hip-width apart. Hold the ball in both hands with the arms straight out in front of you and parallel to the floor. Inhale to begin.
2. Step back approximately 2 feet (0.5 m) with the right foot, toes facing forward.
3. Exhale as you raise the extended arms overhead and flex the left knee to lengthen the right hip.
4. Return to the starting position.
5. Perform 6 to 8 repetitions on each side.

Alignment Cues
- Keep the spine lengthened and in neutral position.
- Lengthen through the anterior hip until you feel a stretch.
- Do not arch the back.
- Move slowly.
- Stay within your range of motion.
- Keep the back heel on the ground and the feet parallel.

Staggered Squat (Ball Between Thighs)

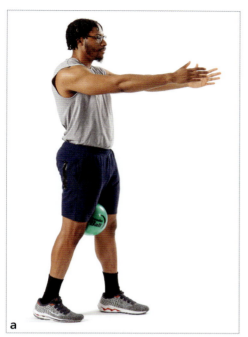
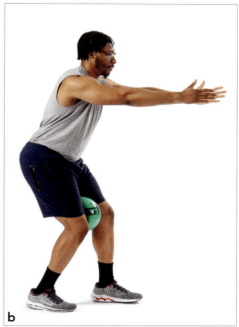

Benefits
The ball helps to align the hips and knees while engaging the adductors and pelvic floor.

Instructions
1. Begin in a staggered position with the right hip posterior (left foot forward) and the ball placed between the thighs.
2. Hold the arms straight out in front of the chest.
3. Placing your weight primarily over the right heel, inhale as you hinge at the hips and flex both knees into a staggered squat.
4. As you lower, extend the spine and feel the right glute and hamstring lengthen.
5. Exhale as you return to standing, engaging the adductors and pelvic floor.
6. Perform 6 to 8 repetitions on each side.

Alignment Cues
- Keep the spine lengthened and in neutral position.
- Do not tuck the pelvis, tighten the glutes, or arch the back.
- Feel the posterior hip doing most of the work.
- Keep your gaze forward.
- Align the knees facing forward and keep the weight over the heels, not the toes.

Parallel Squat (Ball Between Hands)

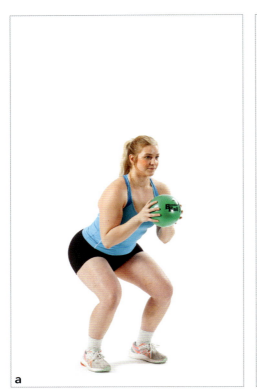
a

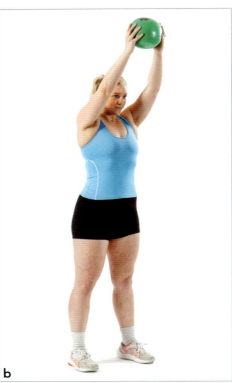
b

Benefits
Putting pressure on the ball with your hands will help you feel the core engage and allow you to gauge range of motion.

Instructions
1. Begin with the feet shoulder-width apart and hold the ball tightly in front of the chest.
2. With the weight over the heels, inhale as you hinge at the hips and flex both knees to lower into a squat.
3. Extend the arms in front of the chest while putting pressure into the ball.
4. Inhale as you lower and exhale as you return to standing, extending the arms overhead.
5. Perform 6 to 8 repetitions.

Alignment Cues
- Keep the spine lengthened and in neutral position.
- Do not tuck the pelvis or tighten the glutes.
- Squat only until you feel the glutes and hamstrings engage.
- Stay within your range of motion.

Variation
Apply more pressure with the right hand and then alternate with the left hand for a different sensation in the core.

Squat With Lateral Flexion and Rotation

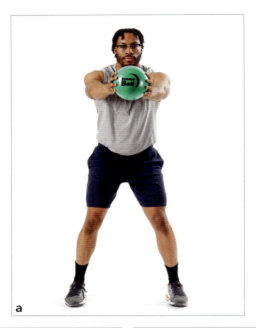

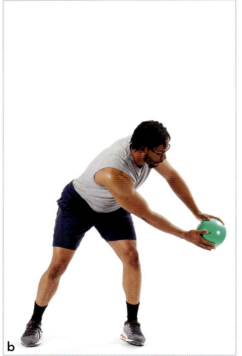

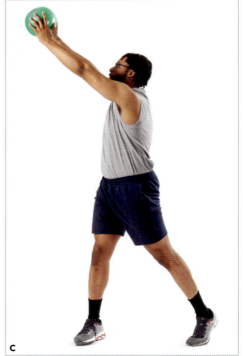

Benefits
The ball helps you gauge the appropriate range of motion and engage the core by adding lateral flexion and rotation against gravity. Holding the ball also enhances alignment.

Instructions
1. Begin with the feet slightly more than hip-width apart and hold the ball in front of the chest.
2. While inhaling, hinge at the hips and flex the knees to lower into a squat while bringing the ball toward the left knee.
3. While exhaling, return to standing while extending the arms overhead and laterally flex the spine to the right.
4. Perform 6 to 8 repetitions on each side.

Alignment Cues
- Make sure to keep the spine lengthened and neutral to engage the core.
- Stay within your range of motion.

Curtsy Lunge With Glider Disc

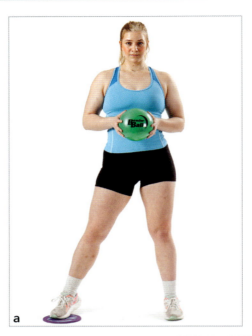
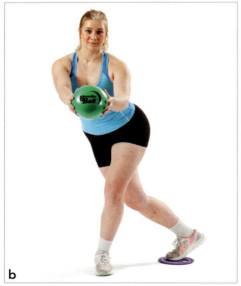
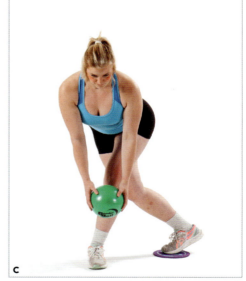

Vertical Exercises 35

Benefits
The ball helps you gauge the appropriate range of motion. Pressing the ball against the thigh will also help activate the core by ensuring better alignment.

Instructions
1. Stand with the feet hip-width apart and hold the ball in both hands in front of the chest.
2. Place the toes of the right foot on the disc.
3. As you inhale, slide the right foot behind you and to your left, rotating the hips while moving the ball toward the left knee.
4. While exhaling, return to the starting position.
5. Perform 6 to 8 repetitions on each side.

Alignment Cues
- Keep the spine lengthened and in neutral position.
- Rotate until you feel the core and glutes engage.
- Stay within your range of motion.
- You can place the ball in between the chest and thigh for alignment assistance and core activation.

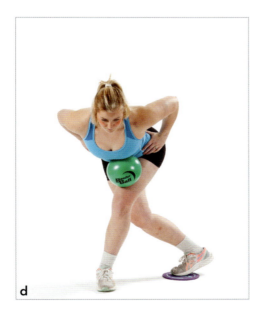
d

Lunge

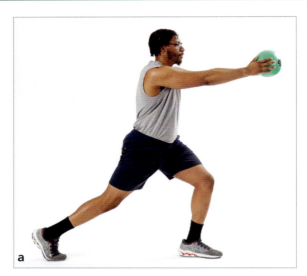

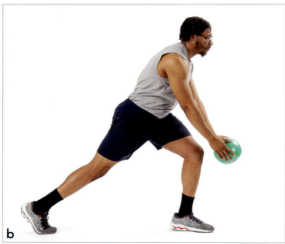

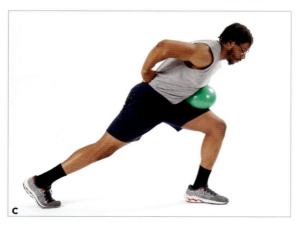

Benefits
This exercise is performed with the ball placed between the thigh and the chest. This helps align the hips and spine and provides core support while keeping the knees over the heels.

Instructions
1. Standing with the feet hip-width apart, step the right foot behind you into a lunge position.
2. Hold the ball in front of the body.
3. Next, reach the ball toward the left knee.
4. Secure the ball in between the left thigh and the chest and place the hands behind the back.
5. Inhale while moving slightly forward until you feel the left glute and core engage.
6. Exhale while moving slightly back until you feel the right glute and core engage.
7. Perform 6 to 8 repetitions on each side.

Alignment Cues
- Keep the spine neutral and hinge from the hips.
- Place the ball where it provides support between the chest and thigh.
- Keep the core engaged to hold the ball in place.
- Keep the front knee in alignment with the heel.
- Focus on engaging and lengthening the glute and hamstring.

Lunge With Glider Disc

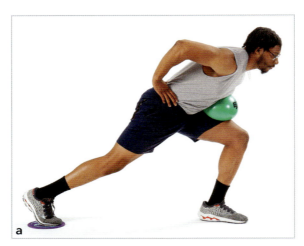

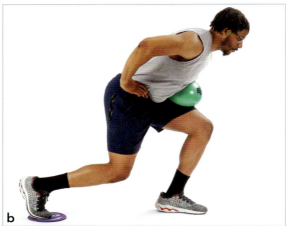

Benefits
This exercise is performed with the ball placed between the thigh and the chest. This helps align the hips and spine and provides core support while keeping the knees over the heels. The glider disc allows the body to move in a fluid range of motion and adds variety to the movement. If a glider disc is not available, you can also use another implement such as a towel or paper plate.

Instructions
1. Standing with the feet hip-width apart, step the right foot behind you into a lunge position and place the glider disc under the toes of the right foot. Hinge forward until the left glute and hamstring are engaged and place the ball between the chest and left thigh. You may reach the arms in front of the body for balance.
2. Inhale to extend the right knee and slide the right foot farther behind you.
3. Exhale to pull the foot toward you and return to the starting position.
4. Perform 6 to 8 repetitions on each side.

Alignment Cues
- Engage the core to keep the ball in place.
- When sliding the back foot, move slowly in order to activate the glutes and hamstrings.
- Keep the front knee aligned over the heel.
- Focus on lengthening the glute and hamstring.

SAFETY TIP Because the back foot is on an unstable surface, move slowly and hold on to a chair or other stable support if needed.

Squat to Balance

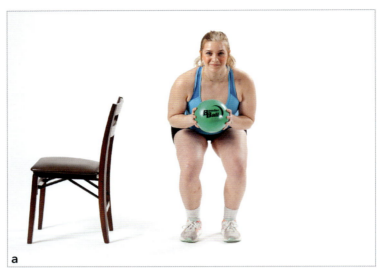

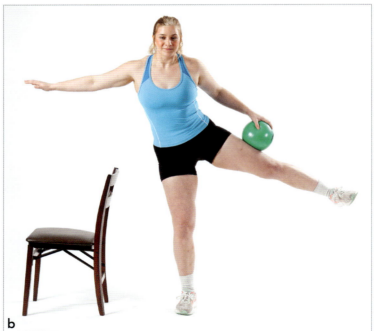

Vertical Exercises 41

Benefits
The ball assists balance, activates the core, and promotes alignment.

Instructions
1. Stand with the feet hip-width apart and hold the ball in both hands.
2. Flex the knees and hips to lower into a squat.
3. Lift and abduct the left hip, straightening the right knee and pressing the ball into the outer left thigh to emphasize engagement of the abductors and core.
4. Hold the balance for 5 seconds while breathing normally.
5. Return to the starting position, then repeat.
6. Perform 6 to 8 repetitions on each side.

Alignment Cues
- Keep the core lengthened and engaged and the spine neutral.
- Do not lift the hip so high that you lose balance.
- Focus on balancing on the supporting leg while abducting the hip.
- Stay within your range of motion.

SAFETY TIP Use a chair or wall for balance if needed.

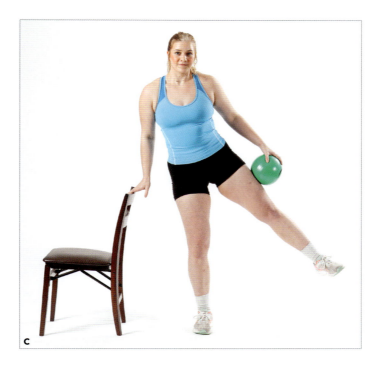
c

Hip Flexion and Balance

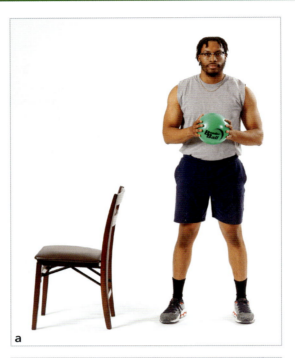

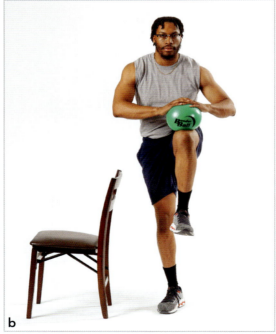

Benefits
The ball provides kinesthetic feedback to gauge range of motion. Pressing into the ball also activates the core.

Instructions
1. Standing with the feet hip-width apart, hold the ball with both hands in front of you at about hip height.
2. Flex the left hip until the knee makes contact with the ball, pressing the knee into the ball until the core engages.
3. Engage the right side of the body for better balance.
4. Hold for approximately 5 seconds while breathing normally.
5. Return to the starting position, then repeat on the other side.
6. Perform 6 to 8 repetitions on each side.

Alignment Cues
- Keep both hips level even when flexing one leg.
- Gently press into the ball for core feedback.
- Focus on balancing on the standing leg.
- Keep the spine neutral.

SAFETY TIP Hold on to a chair to assist with balance if needed.

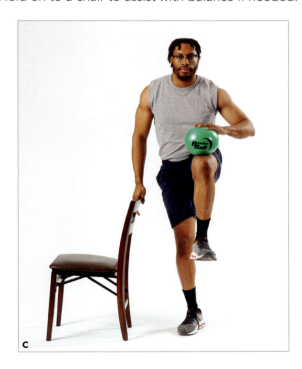
c

Two-Handed Wall Press

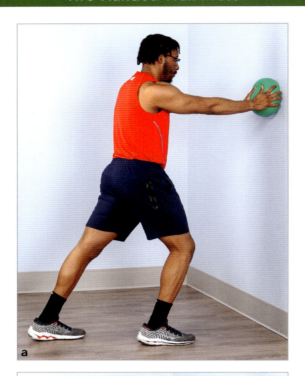

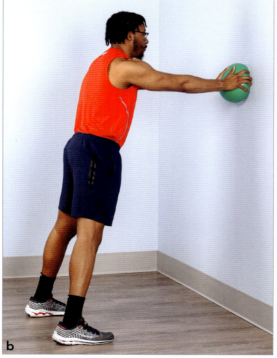

Benefits

Using the ball as an unstable surface provides immediate feedback to the entire core.

Instructions

1. While facing a wall, place the ball against the wall at chest height.
2. Step the right foot forward to establish balance and stability.
3. Alternatively, stand with the feet hip-width apart or narrower for a greater balance challenge.
4. Gently press into the ball with both hands until the core is activated.
5. Hold for 5 seconds, breathing normally.
6. Perform 6 to 8 repetitions.

Alignment Cues

- Activate and depress the scapula area to support the shoulders.
- Do not press so hard into the ball that you create discomfort in the wrists.
- Keep the spine neutral to engage the core and keep the hips wide enough that you can balance.
- Focus on the breath to deepen the core activation.

One-Handed Wall Press

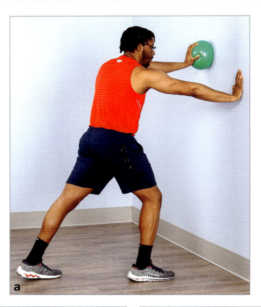

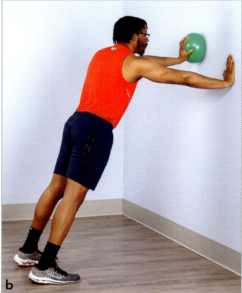

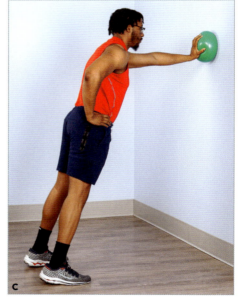

Benefits
Using the ball as an unstable surface under one hand provides immediate feedback to the entire core.

Instructions
1. Using the left hand, place the ball on the wall at chest height and place the right hand on the wall.
2. Step the right foot forward to establish balance and stability.
3. Alternatively, stand with the feet hip-width apart or narrower for a greater balance challenge.
4. Take the right hand off the wall and place it at the side or rest the right hand on the right hip.
5. Roll the ball in various small directions to engage the core for about 5 to 10 seconds, activating and engaging the left side of the body while breathing normally.
6. Perform 6 to 8 repetitions on each side.

Alignment Cues
- Do not press so hard into the ball that you create discomfort in the wrist.
- Keep the spine neutral to engage the core.
- Keep the hips wide enough that you can balance.
- Focus on the breath to deepen the core activation.

Back Press to Wall

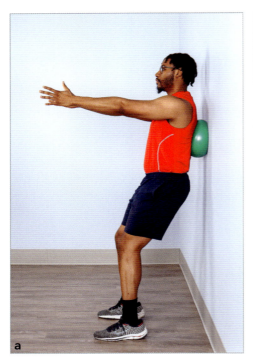 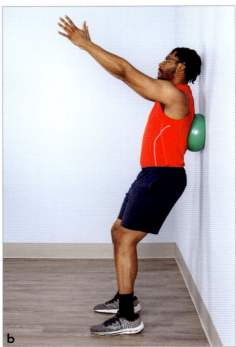

Benefits
The ball provides immediate feedback to the core and supports the spine, which promotes alignment.

Instructions
1. Stand facing away from the wall with the feet hip-width apart and place the ball between the upper back and the wall. Slightly pressing the back into the ball to keep it in place, extend the arms in front of the chest and flex the knees slightly.
2. Inhale with the arms in front of the chest.
3. Exhale and lift the arms slightly above the shoulders.
4. Inhale to extend the arms overhead and extend the spine while gazing upward. Keep the knees soft.
5. Perform 6 to 8 repetitions.

Alignment Cues
- Focus on engaging the core throughout the movement.
- Do not arch the back.
- Keep the knees aligned over the feet.
- Focus on the breath.

Back Press to Wall With Rotation

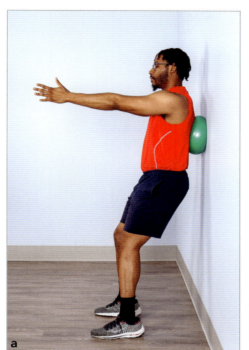 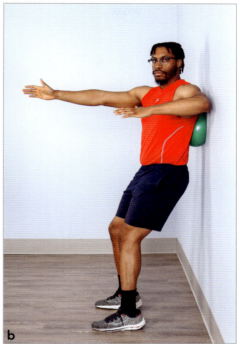

Benefits
The ball provides immediate feedback to the core and supports the spine, which promotes alignment.

Instructions
1. Stand facing away from the wall with the feet hip-width apart and place the ball between the upper back and the wall. Slightly pressing the back into the ball to keep it in place, extend the arms in front of the chest and flex the knees slightly.
2. Inhale with the arms in front of the chest.
3. Exhale and rotate the chest to the left while flexing the left arm to 90 degrees until it touches the wall.
4. Inhale to return to the starting position.
5. Perform 6 to 8 repetitions on each side.

Alignment Cues
- Focus on engaging the core throughout the movement.
- Move slowly through the rotation.
- Keep the knees aligned over the feet.
- Bend the knees slightly more for greater intensity.
- Focus on the breath while rotating the torso.

Lateral Flexion Against the Wall

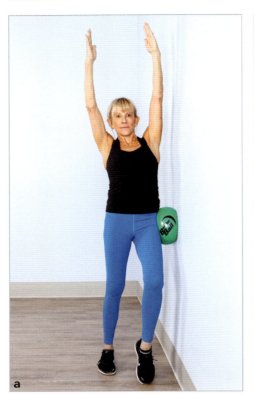 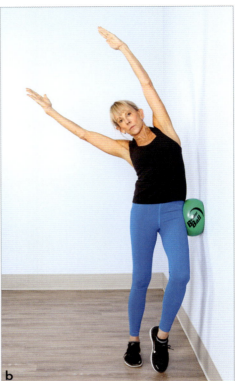

Benefits
Standing next to a wall provides stability and mobility for the spine when laterally flexing to activate the obliques.

Instructions
1. Begin by standing with the left side facing approximately 1 foot (0.3 m) away from the wall.
2. Place the ball on the left hip and press it gently against the wall.
3. Bend the left knee slightly, keeping the toes touching the floor for balance.
4. Inhale while reaching the arms overhead.
5. Exhale while laterally flexing away from the wall.
6. Perform 6 to 8 repetitions on each side of the body.

Alignment Cues
- Make sure to lift and lengthen and not collapse into the spine.
- Only lift the foot off the floor if you can maintain balance.
- Do not rotate the spine.

Variation
For an added balance challenge, flex the knee closest to the wall so the toes are not touching the floor.

Balance (Ball Under Foot)

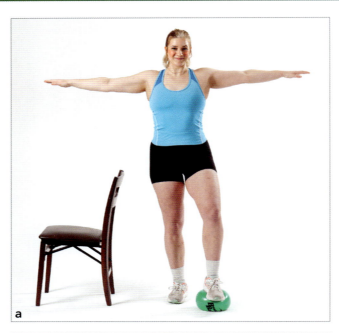

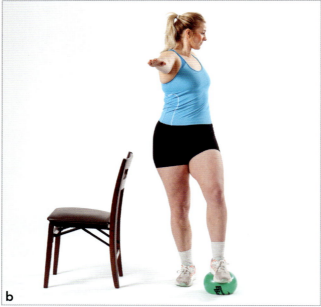

Vertical Exercises 53

Benefits
Having one foot on the ball, an unstable surface, challenges the core.

Instructions
1. While balancing on the right leg, place the ball under the left foot and gently apply pressure. Abduct the arms to the sides for balance and inhale.
2. Exhale as you rotate the torso slowly to the left.
3. Inhale to return to the starting position.
4. Perform 6 to 8 repetitions on each side.

Alignment Cues
- Focus on the supporting side for balance.
- Stand tall and do not apply full body weight on the ball.
- Rotate only until you feel the core engage.
- Focus on the breath through the rotation.

SAFETY TIP   Use a chair or wall for balance if needed.

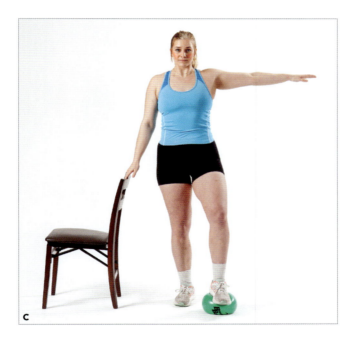

Balance (Ball Inside Knee)

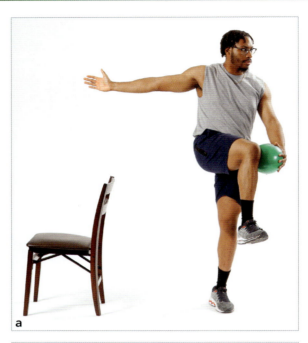

a

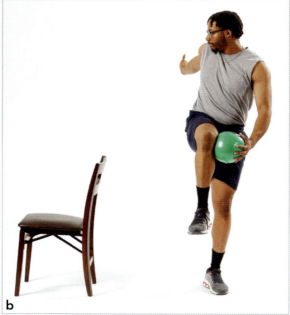

b

Vertical Exercises

Benefits
Pressing the ball to the inside of the knee activates the adductors, which are a part of the deep core muscles, as well as the obliques. It also creates a balance challenge and provides immediate feedback to the core.

Instructions
1. Stand with the feet hip-width apart, holding the ball in the left hand. Flex the right hip to bring the right foot off the floor in front of you and press the ball into the right inner thigh above the knee.
2. Keeping the spine lifted and lengthened, inhale to initiate rotation of the upper body to the left.
3. Exhale as you rotate to the right.
4. Return to the starting position.
5. Perform 6 to 8 repetitions on each side.

Alignment Cues
- Focus on balancing on the supporting leg.
- Gently press the hand into the ball to engage the core.

SAFETY TIP Use a chair or wall for balance if needed.

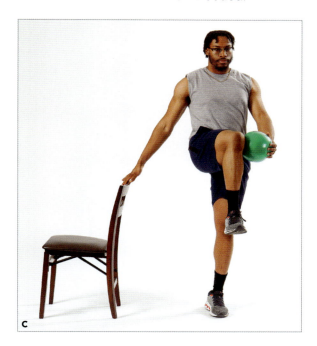

Balance (Ball Outside Knee)

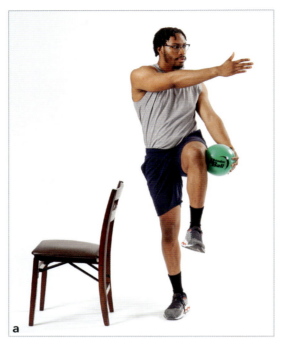

a

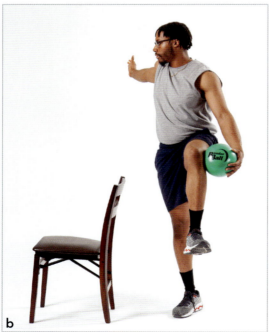

b

Vertical Exercises

Benefits
Pressing the ball to the outside of the knee activates the outer abductors and obliques. It also creates a balance challenge and provides immediate feedback to the core.

Instructions
1. Stand with the feet hip-width apart, holding the ball in the left hand. Flex the left hip to bring the left foot off the floor in front of you and press the ball into the outside of the left thigh just above the knee.
2. Keep the spine lifted and lengthened.
3. Inhale as you initiate rotation of the upper body to the left.
4. Exhale as you rotate to the right.
5. Return to the starting position.
6. Perform 6 to 8 repetitions on each side.

Alignment Cues
- Focus on balancing on the supporting leg.
- Gently press the hand into the ball to engage the core.

SAFETY TIP Use a chair or wall for balance if needed.

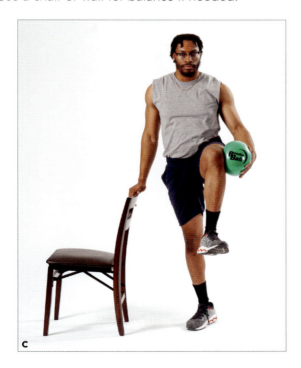
c

CHAPTER 4

Kneeling Exercises

In this chapter you will learn how to train the core using the ball in kneeling exercises. The ball can provide slight instability in specific exercises to challenge the body's core, and it can also give support under the knee(s) or hand(s), especially for those who have knee pain or discomfort. Performing effective exercises in a kneeling position also strengthens the upper extremities such as the shoulder complex as you use body weight against gravity. When initiating any of the movements, it is important to keep the spine neutral and the body's core slightly engaged so that breathing is not inhibited.

It is important to allow the client to find the best position using regressions and progressions. Many clients with wrist or knee issues find any kneeling or planking painful, but with the ball and good alignment, most exercises can be performed successfully. Ensuring good alignment and not allowing the back or shoulders to arch is crucial. The more the body adapts to correct alignment, the more it becomes second nature, especially in a kneeling position. The body will become stronger in practice, and then you can help clients move on to more difficult positions and movements.

The exercises and stretches are color coded. Exercises in green are for all levels of participants. Exercises in blue are slightly more challenging yet appropriate for most participants. Exercises in red are for higher-level participants looking for a more challenging exercise.

You will find that most of the exercises in this text are suitable for everyone. However, if an exercise seems too difficult, then alignment or outcome can be compromised; therefore, make sure the exercise feels good to the client's body so the goal can be achieved. Keep in mind that good alignment and form are more important than anything else with all exercises in this program.

Benefits and Cues

Using the ball with kneeling exercises provides several benefits. The small ball can

- help align the hips,
- add stability by engaging the inner thighs,
- add a visual aid, and
- provide cushioning under the knees or hands.

The following alignment cues should be reviewed before undertaking the exercises:

- Keep the spine neutral and the core slightly engaged at all times *(a)*.
- Keep the gaze down or slightly forward to prevent neck strain *(b)*.
- Lift off of the wrists.
- Do not let the spine or shoulders arch, creating pressure or discomfort *(c)*.
- Move slowly and deliberately with the intention of achieving the desired outcome.
- Breathe to increase mobility in the core.
- Do not squeeze the ball so much that it creates dysfunctional posture.
- Do not put full body weight on the ball.

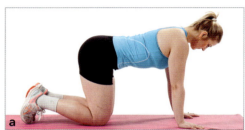
a

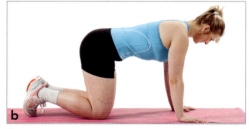
b

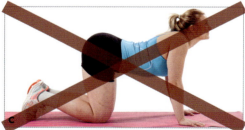
c

Kneeling (Ball Between Thighs)

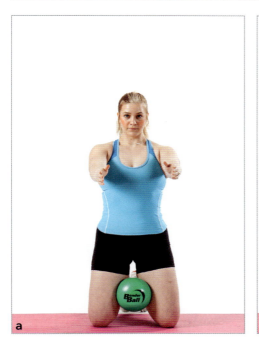
a

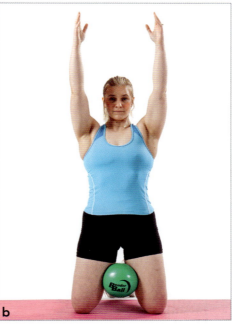
b

Benefits
Kneeling with the ball between the thighs while reaching the arms overhead activates the deep pelvic floor muscles and obliques.

Instructions
1. Kneel on a padded surface with the ball between the thighs and the arms extended in front of you.
2. Inhale to initiate with the arms in front of the chest.
3. Exhale and reach the arms above the shoulders.
4. Return to the starting position while lifting the body.
5. Perform 6 to 8 repetitions.

Alignment Cues
- Keep the spine neutral.
- Engage the inner thighs, core, and pelvic floor as you reach the arms above the shoulders.
- Keep the shoulders down and relaxed.
- Do not arch the back.
- Keep your gaze slightly upward.

Variation
Engage the right thigh by pressing it slightly into the ball; repeat with the left thigh for a different feeling in the core.

Kneeling With Lateral Flexion (Ball Between Thighs)

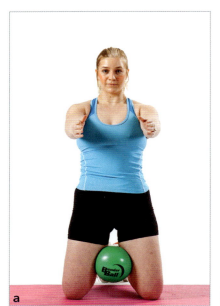 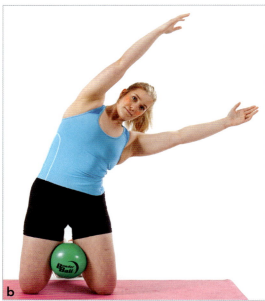

Benefits
Kneeling with the ball between the thighs while alternating lateral flexion engages the deep pelvic floor muscles and obliques. Working against gravity while flexing also engages the obliques as part of the core.

Instructions
1. Kneel on a padded surface with the ball between the thighs.
2. Lift through the torso.
3. Inhale to initiate, raising the arms overhead.
4. As you exhale, laterally flex the torso to the left and engage the right inner thigh.
5. Inhale to return to the starting position, then repeat on the other side.
6. Perform 6 to 8 repetitions on each side.

Kneeling Exercises **63**

Alignment Cues
- Keep the spine neutral.
- Engage the muscles of the inner thighs that affect the deep core muscles.
- Keep your gaze forward to maintain balance.
- Laterally flex only until you feel the obliques and core engage.

SAFETY TIP If you have trouble keeping upright without tipping forward, place your hands on your hips.

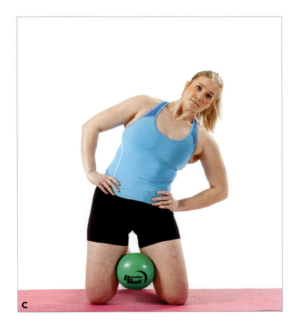

Kneeling With Rotation (Ball Between Thighs)

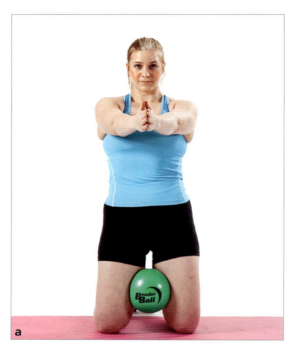

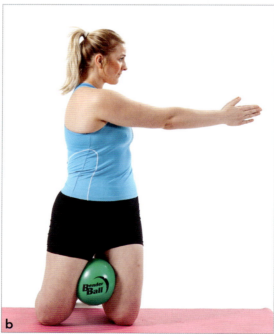

Benefits
Kneeling with the ball between the thighs while rotating engages the deep pelvic floor muscles and obliques. Although gravity is not an influence, pure rotation comes from the obliques as part of the core.

Instructions
1. Kneel on a padded surface with the ball between the thighs and the arms extended at shoulder height in front of you, hands together.
2. Inhale to initiate with the arms in front of the body.
3. While exhaling, slowly rotate the torso to the left and engage the right inner thigh.
4. Inhale to return to the starting position, then repeat on the other side.
5. Perform 6 to 8 repetitions on each side.

Alignment Cues
- Lift the torso off of the hips.
- Think of lengthening when rotating.
- Only rotate until you feel the core and inner thighs engage.
- Apply only light pressure to the ball with the thighs.
- Allow your gaze to follow the direction of rotation, letting the head and neck rotate with the torso.

Kneeling With Knee Lifts (Ball Between Knees)

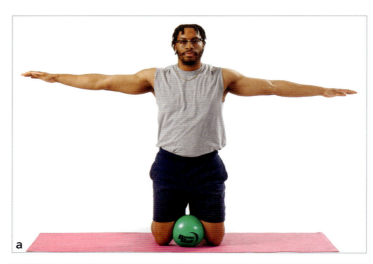

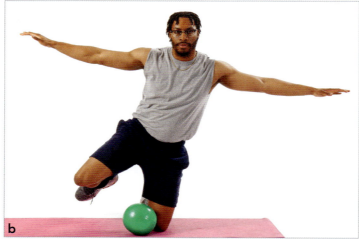

Benefits
Balancing on the knees challenges the body's core differently than balancing on the feet. It is a greater balance challenge than simply taking a foot off of the floor.

Instructions
1. Kneel on a padded surface with the ball between the knees and the arms extended at the sides for balance.
2. Slightly lift the right knee off of the floor a few inches for about 3 to 5 seconds. Continue to breathe normally.
3. Return to the starting position, then repeat on the other side.
4. Perform 6 to 8 repetitions on each side.

Alignment Cues
- Focus on lengthening the body to activate the core.
- Do not lift the knee so high that you lose balance.
- Keep your gaze forward.

Variations
For a regression, only place the ball under one knee, which does not require as much balance. For an added balance challenge, rotate the head in the same direction as the raised knee.

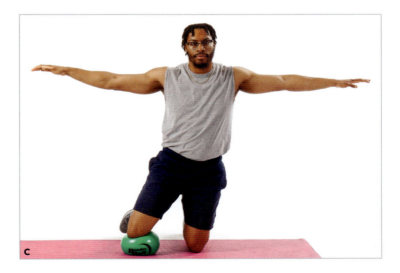

Hands and Knees (Ball Under Hand)

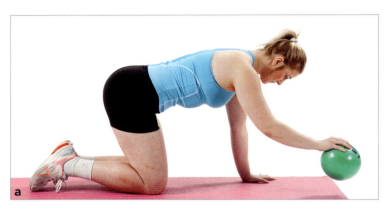

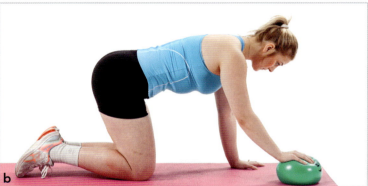

Benefits
Placing the ball under one hand creates instability and provides feedback to the body's core.

Instructions
1. Kneeling on the hands and knees on a padded surface, align the knees under the hips and the left hand under the shoulder. Place the right hand on the ball, slightly in front of the left hand.
2. Slightly press into the ball for 5 seconds, breathing normally.
3. Perform 6 to 8 repetitions on each side, either by alternating or performing all repetitions on one side before switching to the other.

Alignment Cues
- Stabilize and engage the supporting wrist and shoulder.
- Apply only light pressure to the ball with the hand.
- Focus on engaging the core as you press slightly into the ball.
- Keep the cervical, thoracic, and lumbar spine neutral.
- Keep your gaze toward the floor.

Hands and Knees With Hip Extension (Ball Under Hand)

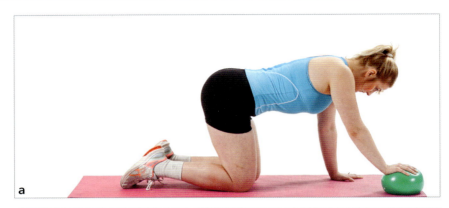

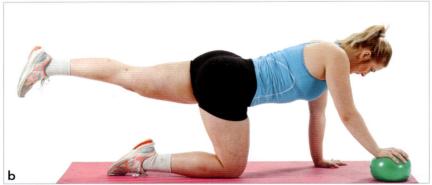

Benefits
Having the ball under one hand with the opposite hip extended creates a greater challenge for the body's core.

Instructions
1. Kneeling on the hands and knees on a padded surface, align the knees under the hips and the left hand under the shoulder. Place the right hand on the ball, slightly in front of the left hand.
2. Gently press the right hand into the ball.
3. Extend the left hip until the left leg is parallel to the floor and even with the hips.
4. Hold for 5 seconds, breathing normally.
5. Return the knee to the floor and repeat on the same side, or alternate to the other side.
6. Perform 6 to 8 repetitions on each side.

Alignment Cues
- Stabilize and lift from the supporting wrist, shoulder, and hip.
- Do not press hard on the ball when lifting the opposite hip.
- Keep the cervical, thoracic, and lumbar spine neutral, especially when extending the hip.
- Keep your gaze toward the floor.
- Move slowly to feel the core engage.

Hands and Knees With Hip Extension (Ball Under Knee)

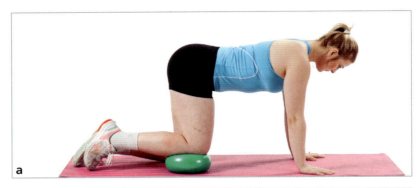

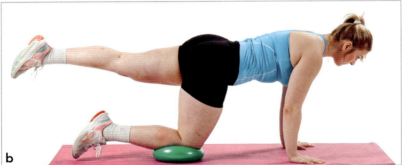

Benefits
Placing the ball under one knee creates instability and provides feedback to the body's core.

Instructions
1. Kneeling on the hands and knees on a padded surface, align the hands directly under the shoulders and place the ball under the right kneecap.
2. Keep the toes of the right foot flexed for stability.
3. Extend the left hip slowly until the left leg is parallel to the floor and even with the hips. Hold for 5 seconds, breathing normally.
4. Return the left knee to the floor and repeat on the same side, or alternate to the other side.
5. Perform 6 to 8 repetitions on each side.

Alignment Cues
- Make sure the ball is positioned securely under the kneecap and the toes are flexed on the floor to provide stability.
- Keep the cervical, thoracic, and lumbar spine neutral.
- Extend the hip only until it is parallel with the body.
- Keep your gaze toward the floor.
- Move slowly to feel the core engage.

Kneeling Exercises 73

Hands and Knees With Glider Disc (Ball Between Thighs)

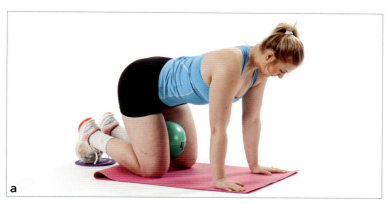

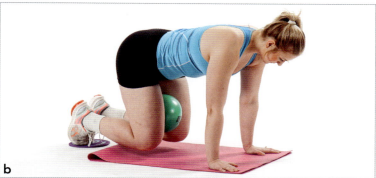

Benefits
This exercise engages the deep pelvic floor muscles and adductors while strengthening the shoulder complex.

Instructions
1. Kneel on the hands and knees on a padded surface with the ball between the thighs, the toes on a glider disc, and the hands aligned directly under the shoulders.
2. Lift the knees to hover slightly off the mat.
3. Hold for 5 seconds, breathing normally.
4. Return to the starting position.
5. Perform 6 to 8 repetitions.

Alignment Cues
- Keep the spine neutral.
- Lift the knees only slightly off the floor, keeping the hips and spine in alignment.
- Move slowly and engage the core and adductors as you lift.
- Keep your gaze toward the floor.

Hands and Knees With Hip Mobility With Glider Disc (Ball Between Thighs)

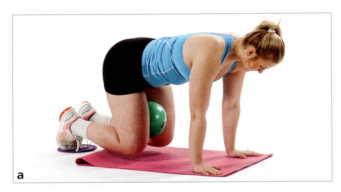

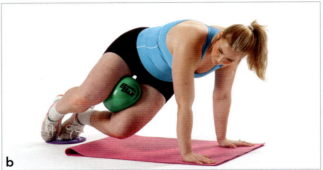

Benefits
This exercise engages the deep pelvic floor muscles, adductors, and obliques while strengthening the shoulder complex.

Instructions
1. Kneel on the hands and knees on a padded surface with the ball between the thighs, the toes on a glider disc, and the hands aligned directly under the shoulders.
2. Inhale to initiate, lifting the knees to hover slightly off the floor.
3. Exhale with good control while slowly swinging the knees to the right.
4. Return to the starting position and repeat on the left side.
5. Inhale to return the knees to the floor.
6. Perform 6 to 8 repetitions on each side.

Alignment Cues
- Engage the core and adductors as you lift and the obliques as the hips move.
- Engage the shoulders to take pressure off the wrists.
- Keep the cervical, thoracic, and lumbar spine neutral.
- Lift the knees only slightly off the floor.
- Keep your gaze toward the floor.

Hands and Knees With Toe Lifts (Ball Between Thighs)

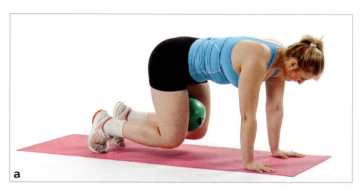

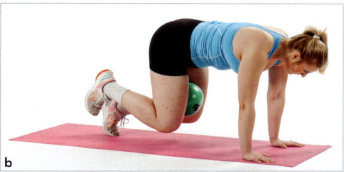

Benefits
This exercise engages the deep core muscles with an added balance challenge.

Instructions
1. Kneel on the hands and knees on a padded surface with the hands aligned directly under the shoulders, the ball between the thighs, the toes tucked under, and the knees hovering off the floor.
2. Inhale to initiate, lifting the right foot off the floor.
3. Exhale and return to the starting position.
4. Repeat on the other side.
5. Perform 6 to 8 repetitions on each side.

Alignment Cues
- Keep the hips level while alternating toe lifts.
- Only lift the foot slightly off of the floor.
- Keep the spine neutral.

Variations
Return both knees to the floor between repetitions if needed or keep them hovering for a greater challenge.

Hands and Knees (Ball Under Knees)

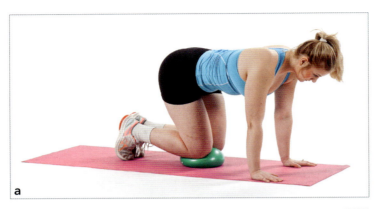

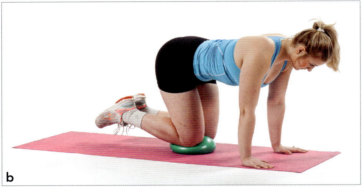

Benefits
Placing the ball under both knees provides a greater balance challenge to the core.

Instructions
1. Kneel on the hands and knees with the kneecaps resting on the ball, the toes tucked under, and the hands aligned directly under the shoulders.
2. Inhale to initiate, lifting the toes of both feet off the mat.
3. Exhale to return to the starting position.
4. Perform 6 to 8 repetitions.

Alignment Cues
- Keep the spine neutral.
- Draw the abdominals in to assist balance.

Variation
Alternate lifting the right and left toes off of the floor.

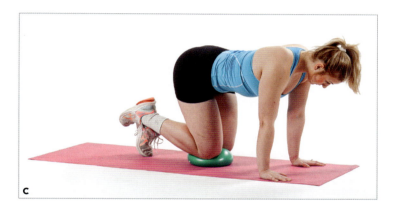

c

CHAPTER 5

Prone Exercises

In this chapter you will learn how to train the core using the small ball in exercises performed face down (prone). In this position, the ball can provide better alignment and core awareness while also aligning the hips and engaging the deep pelvic floor muscles.

Engaging the upper extremities as well as the lower benefits the entire body, which means you can perform a smaller number of repetitions while still achieving benefits. All the exercises in this chapter are to be performed slowly and with intention to fully work the muscles in the core and help to protect the back from the risk of injury. When initiating any of the movements, it is important to keep the spine neutral and the core slightly engaged so that breathing is not inhibited.

The exercises and stretches are color coded. Exercises in green are for all levels of participants. Exercises in blue are slightly more challenging yet appropriate for most participants. Exercises in red are for higher-level participants looking for a more challenging exercise.

You will find that most of the exercises in this text are suitable for everyone. However, if an exercise seems too difficult, then alignment or outcome can be compromised; therefore, make sure the exercise feels good to the client's body so the goal can be achieved. Keep in mind that good alignment and form are more important than anything else with all exercises in this program.

Benefits and Cues

Using the ball with prone exercises provides several benefits. The small ball can
- help align the hips and
- give kinesthetic feedback to help maintain good alignment and posture.

The following alignment cues should be reviewed before undertaking the exercises:
- Make sure to place the ball in the correct position for proper alignment *(a)*.
- Keep the spine neutral to protect the back *(b)*.
- Do not let the low back or shoulders drop *(c)*.
- Always lower the knees for regression of any exercise.
- Move slowly and deliberately with the intention of achieving the desired outcome.

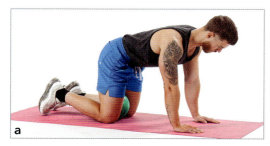

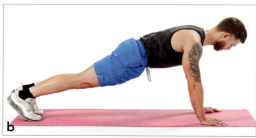

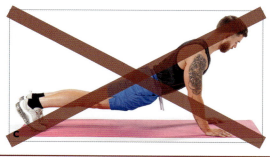

Forearm Plank (Ball Under Chest)

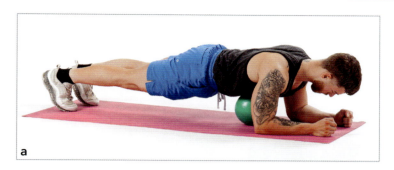

Benefits
Placing the ball under the chest keeps the body in alignment and the spine neutral. It also provides kinesthetic feedback.

Instructions
1. Begin on the knees and forearms on a padded surface, placing the ball directly under the chest. Make sure the forearms are aligned directly under the shoulders.
2. Lift one knee off the floor, then the other.
3. Hold the plank for 5 seconds, breathing normally.
4. Keep the chest hovering lightly over the ball, just touching it.
5. Return to the starting position, then repeat.
6. Perform 6 to 8 repetitions.

Alignment Cues
- Keep the cervical spine neutral.
- Use the ball as feedback to check on your alignment (imagine you are floating the chest just over the ball).
- Do not arch the back or let the hips collapse.
- Keep your gaze forward.

Variation
Alternate lifting the right and left knee off of the floor.

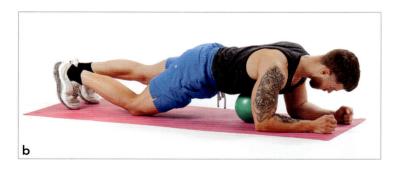

Forearm Plank With Hip Extension (Ball Under Chest)

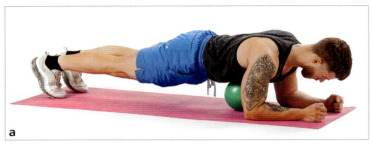

a

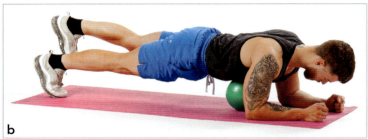

b

Benefits
Placing the ball under the chest keeps the body in alignment and the spine neutral. It also provides kinesthetic feedback.

Instructions
1. Begin on the knees and forearms on a padded surface, placing the ball directly under the chest. Make sure the forearms are aligned directly under the shoulders.
2. Start with one knee off of the floor to find alignment.
3. Lift both knees off of the floor to a full plank.
4. Lift the left foot off of the floor and extend the hip.
5. Hold for 5 seconds, breathing normally.
6. Keep the chest hovering lightly over the ball, just touching it.
7. Return to the starting position, then repeat on the other side.
8. Perform 6 to 8 repetitions on each side.

Alignment Cues
- Keep the cervical spine neutral.
- Use the ball as feedback to check on your alignment (imagine you are floating the chest just over the ball).
- Do not arch the back or let the hips collapse.
- Keep your gaze forward.

Variation
For a regression, return the knees to the floor between leg lifts.

Plank (Ball Between Thighs)

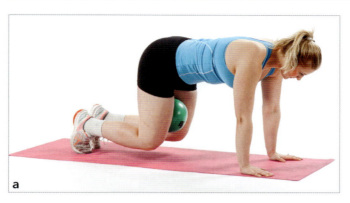

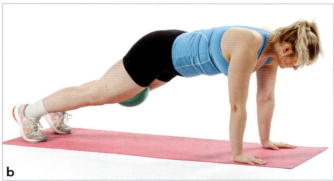

Benefits
Planking with the ball between the thighs keeps the hips aligned and engages the deep pelvic floor muscles.

Instructions
1. Begin on the hands and knees on a padded surface, with the hands directly under the shoulders, the knees directly under the hips, and the ball between the thighs.
2. Lift the knees off the mat and move into a plank position, with the toes, knees, hips, and shoulders in one long line.
3. Hold for 5 seconds, engaging the inner thighs and breathing normally.
4. Return to the starting position.
5. Perform 6 to 8 repetitions.

Alignment Cues
- Keep the cervical, thoracic, and lumbar spine neutral.
- Engage the adductors and the deep core muscles.
- Do not let the lower back or hips drop.
- Keep your gaze forward.

Plank With Hip Extension (Ball Between Thighs)

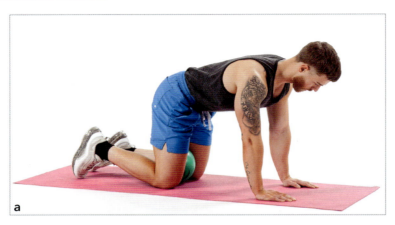

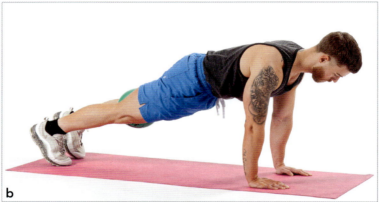

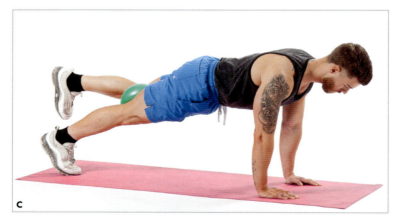

Benefits
Planking with the ball between the thighs keeps the hips aligned and engages the deep pelvic floor muscles. Extending one hip also requires better overall core control.

Instructions
1. Begin on the hands and knees on a padded surface, with the hands directly under the shoulders, the knees directly under the hips, and the ball between the thighs.
2. Lift the knees off the mat and move into a plank position, with the toes, knees, hips, and shoulders in one long line.
3. Extend the left hip and lift the left foot off of the mat, engaging the left inner thigh.
4. Hold for 5 seconds, breathing normally.
5. Lower the knees, then repeat on the other side.
6. Perform 6 to 8 repetitions on each side.

Alignment Cues
- Keep the cervical, thoracic, and lumbar spine neutral.
- Keep the hips level as you lift the foot.
- Move slowly and engage the deep pelvic floor muscles and adductors.
- Keep your gaze forward.

Plank With Rotation (Ball Between Thighs)

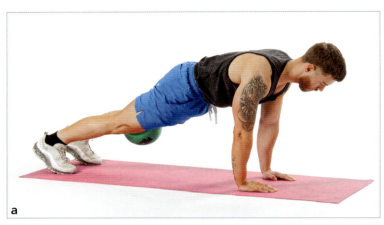

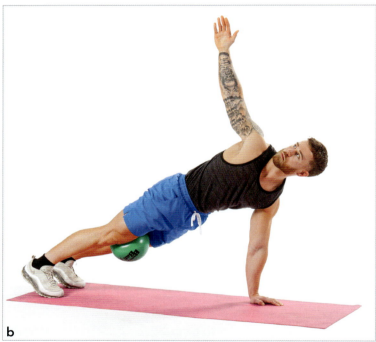

Benefits
Planking with the ball between the thighs keeps the hips aligned and engages the deep pelvic floor muscles while strengthening the upper extremities. The rotation engages both the upper body and obliques simultaneously.

Instructions
1. Begin on the hands and knees on a padded surface with the hands directly under the shoulders, the knees directly under the hips, and the ball between the thighs.
2. Inhale to initiate and lift the knees off the mat.
3. Exhale and rotate the torso, lifting the right hand off of the mat.
4. Extend the right arm toward the ceiling.
5. Return to the starting position.
6. Repeat on the same side or alternate sides.
7. Perform 6 to 8 repetitions on each side.

Alignment Cues
- Keep the cervical spine neutral.
- Engage the adductors for core support.
- Move slowly and with intention.
- Keep your gaze upward as you lift and rotate through the body.

Variation
As a regression, keep both knees on the mat while rotating through the spine.

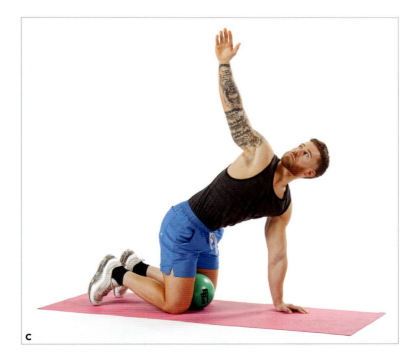
c

Plank to Pike With Glider Disc (Ball Between Thighs)

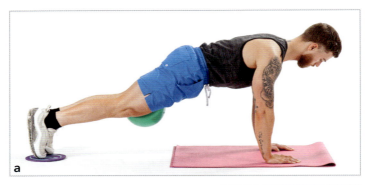

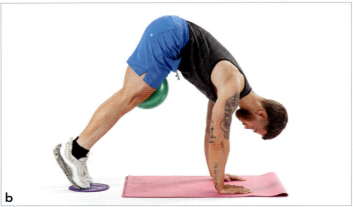

Benefits
Planking with the ball between the thighs keeps the hips aligned and activates the deep pelvic floor muscles.

Instructions
1. Begin on the hands and knees on a padded surface with the hands directly under the shoulders and the toes on a glider disc.
2. Inhale to initiate, then lift the knees and slide the feet back into a plank.
3. Exhale, then lift the hips into a pike position.
4. Return to the starting position, moving fluidly.
5. Return to a plank or lower the knees to rest on the mat, then repeat.
6. Perform 6 to 8 repetitions.

Alignment Cues
- Keep the cervical, thoracic, and lumbar spine neutral.
- Lift the hips only as high as is comfortable, especially if the hamstrings are tight and limit motion.
- Move slowly and engage the deep pelvic floor muscles.
- Keep your gaze forward.

Prone Exercises 89

Forearm Plank With Hip Rotation With Glider Disc (Ball Between Thighs)

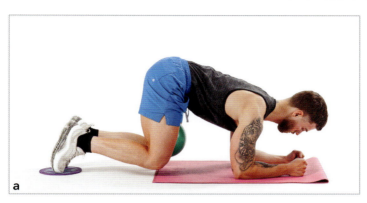

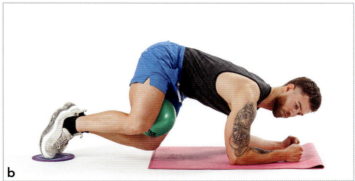

Benefits
Performing this movement with the ball between the thighs will keep the hips aligned while rotating and engaging the deep core muscles.

Instructions
1. Begin on the knees and forearms on a padded surface with the ball between the thighs.
2. Place the feet on the glider disc.
3. Inhale to initiate, hovering the knees off of the mat.
4. Exhale, rotating the hips and knees to the right.
5. Lower the knees to the floor, then repeat on the same side or alternate sides.
6. Perform 6 to 8 repetitions on each side.

Alignment Cues
- Keep the spine extended throughout.
- Rotate only until you feel the obliques engage.
- Engage the adductors and obliques.

Forearm Plank (Ball Between Hands)

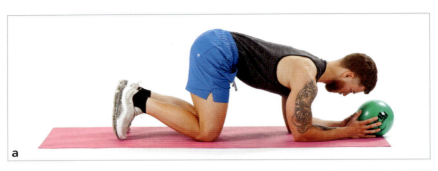

a

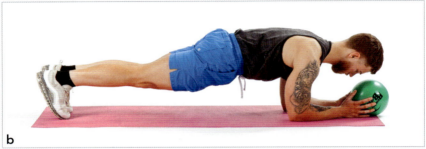

b

Benefits
Planking with the ball between the hands keeps the shoulders and upper extremities aligned.

Instructions
1. Begin on the knees and forearms on a padded surface with the ball between the hands.
2. Place pressure on the ball, lift the knees off of the mat, and step the feet back, breathing normally.
3. Hold for 5 seconds.
4. Return to the starting position, then repeat.
5. Perform 6 to 8 repetitions.

Alignment Cues
- Keep the cervical, thoracic, and lumbar spine neutral.
- Engage the core when lifting the knees off the floor.
- Do not apply too much pressure to the ball; only squeeze enough to engage the core.

Prone Spinal Extension (Ball Under Hands)

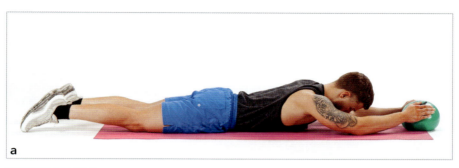

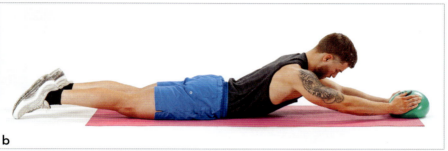

Benefits
The ball provides a softer surface underneath the hands and slight elevation of the shoulders and thoracic spine.

Instructions
1. Begin in a prone position on a padded surface with the arms extended overhead and both hands placed on the ball, keeping slight flexion in the elbows.
2. Inhale to initiate and press slightly into the ball. Lift the torso, keeping the thighs on the floor.
3. Move fluidly.
4. Exhale to return to the starting position, then repeat.
5. Perform 6 to 8 repetitions.

Alignment Cues
- Keep the cervical spine neutral.
- Do not lift the hips.
- Lift the torso only until you feel the back and shoulders engage.
- Think of lengthening the spine rather than lifting the torso higher.
- Keep the shoulder blades down.
- Engage the deep core muscles.

Prone Hip Extension (Ball Between Ankles)

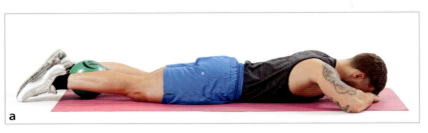

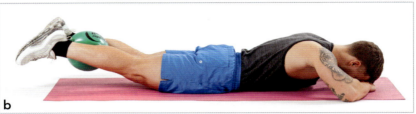

Benefits
Prone hip extension strengthens the back core muscles and glutes, which are important in posture and alignment.

Instructions
1. Begin in a prone position on a padded surface with the forehead on the hands. The ball is between the ankles and the legs are parallel.
2. Inhale to initiate.
3. Exhale to lift the thighs slightly off the mat while engaging the glutes.
4. Lower the legs back to the mat.
5. Move fluidly while repeating the movement.
6. Perform 6 to 8 repetitions.

Alignment Cues
- Move slowly and think of lifting the abdominals off the mat.
- Engage the glutes, posterior core muscles, and inner thighs.
- Do not arch the back.
- Do not lift more than a couple of inches off the ground.
- Do not lift the head off the hands.

SAFETY TIP You can place a towel under the forehead for support.

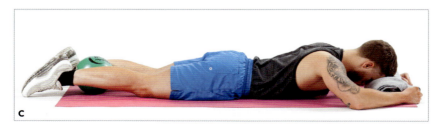

CHAPTER 6

Side-Lying Exercises

In this chapter you will learn how to use the ball to laterally flex and extend the torso and activate the core and obliques. It is important to place the ball so that it supports the body and encourages good alignment so that you do not feel the exercise in the lower back. It is also important to keep the bottom hip flexed in front of the body for good alignment and support. To perform an exercise most effectively, hold the head so the cervical spine is in alignment. Using a glider disc will help ensure smooth movement when performing these side-lying exercises. If you experience any neck or back discomfort, either adjust how your body is positioned or consider only using the vertical exercises in chapter 3.

The exercises and stretches are color coded. Exercises in green are for all levels of participants. Exercises in blue are slightly more challenging yet appropriate for most participants. Exercises in red are for higher-level participants looking for a more challenging exercise.

You will find that most of the exercises in this text are suitable for everyone. However, if an exercise seems too difficult, then alignment or outcome can be compromised; therefore, make sure the exercise feels good to the client's body so the goal can be achieved. Keep in mind that good alignment and form are more important than anything else with all exercises in this program.

Benefits and Cues

Using the ball with side-lying exercises provides several benefits. The small ball can

- provide kinesthetic feedback to the lateral core,
- provide support for body weight, and
- allow for lateral flexion and extension.

The following alignment cues should be reviewed before undertaking the exercises:

- Make sure that the ball is positioned between the ribs and hip (under the rib cage). The position might be slightly different for longer or shorter torsos *(a)*.
- Make sure that the body is aligned comfortably on the ball *(b)*.
- Flex the bottom hip for balance when necessary.

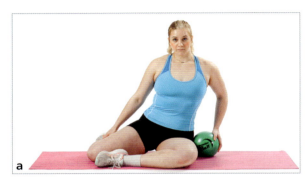

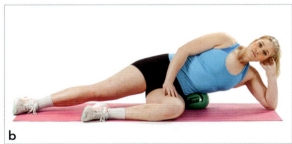

Side-Lying Lateral Flexion (Ball Under Side)

Benefits
The position of the ball allows the spine to laterally flex and engage the obliques while protecting the back and neck.

Instructions
1. Begin by lying on the left side with the left elbow on the mat and the left hand supporting the head. Place the ball in between the ribs and hip.
2. Bring the right hand to the mat in front of the chest.
3. Flex the left hip and knee in front of the body for stability.
4. Inhale to initiate, lifting the left elbow off of the mat while keeping the right hand in front of the body.

Side-Lying Exercises   95

5. Exhale slowly and laterally flex the spine.
6. Moving fluidly, return to the starting position, then repeat.
7. Perform 6 to 8 repetitions on each side.

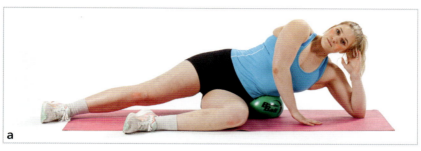

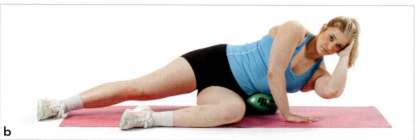

Alignment Cues
- Keep the cervical spine neutral.
- Lift the elbow off the floor only until the obliques engage.
- Move slowly so as not to strain the neck.
- Keep the top hip parallel to the body so as not to place any pressure on the low back.
- Keep your gaze forward.

Variations
For a greater core challenge, take the top hand off of the mat and keep it to the side of the body or raise the top arm to the ceiling as you flex the spine.

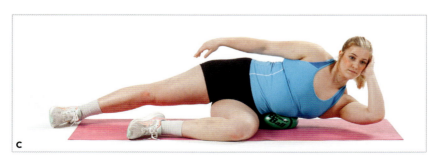

Side-Lying Lateral Flexion With Glider Disc (Ball Under Side)

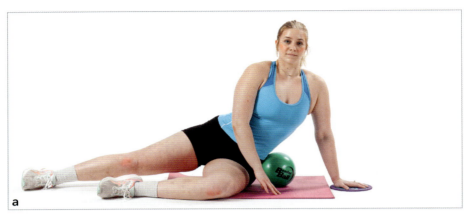

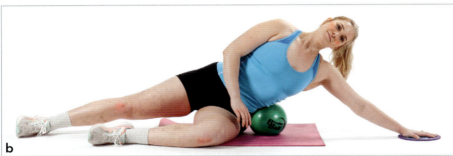

Benefits
Combining the ball and a glider disc to execute the movement allows for greater lengthening of the side of the body. If a glider disc is not available, you can also use another implement such as a towel or paper plate.

Instructions
1. Begin by sitting on the left side of the body on a mat with the left hand on the glider disc. The arm should be aligned with the left shoulder.
2. Secure the ball next to the left hip and place the right hand in front or to the side of the body.
3. The right leg should be straight and aligned to the side of the body.
4. Keep the left hip flexed in front of the body for support.
5. Inhale to initiate, laterally lengthening to the left and sliding the disc slightly away from the body.
6. Moving fluidly, exhale to slide the hand back to the starting position.
7. Perform 6 to 8 repetitions on each side.

Alignment Cues
- Press the hand into the glider disc to lift the body and engage the obliques.
- Think of lengthening the body when sliding the hand and shoulder away from the body.
- Lift the torso only until the obliques engage.
- Keep the hand slightly at an angle so as not to impinge the shoulder.
- Move slowly so as not to strain the neck or back.

Variation
Reach the top arm to the side of the body for an additional challenge.

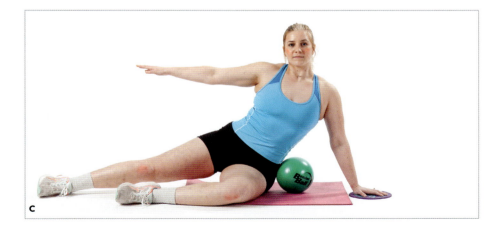

c

Side-Lying Hip Adduction (Ball Between Ankles)

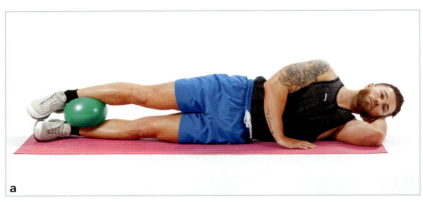

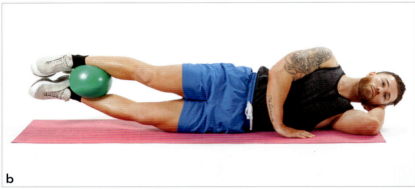

Benefits
The ball assists in engaging the adductors, which can affect pelvic floor function and strength.

Instructions
1. Begin by lying on a padded surface on the left side with the head resting on the left forearm or a towel and the ball between the ankles.
2. Inhale to initiate and engage the inner thighs.
3. Exhale and lift the legs off of the mat.
4. Moving fluidly, lower the legs to the floor, then repeat.
5. Perform 6 to 8 repetitions on each side.

Alignment Cues
- Keep the cervical spine neutral.
- Lift the hips only slightly off the floor.
- Move slowly to engage the inner thighs.
- Imagine lengthening the body throughout the movement.
- Keep your gaze forward.

SAFETY TIP   Place a towel under the head for support.

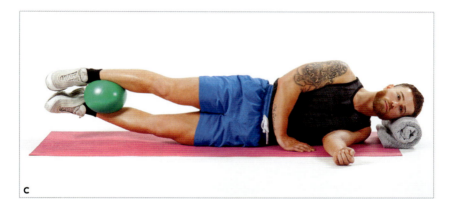

c

Forearm Side Plank (Ball Between Thighs)

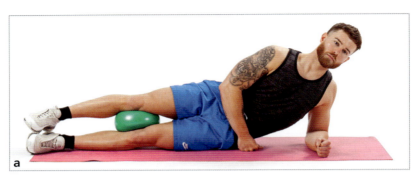

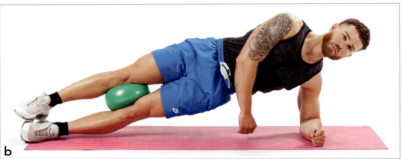

Side-Lying Exercises

Benefits
The ball assists in engaging the adductors and deep core muscles.

Instructions
1. Begin by lying on a padded surface on the left side with the upper body supported on the forearm, the hips and knees straight, and the ball between the thighs.
2. Lift the hips off of the floor and engage the inner thighs.
3. Hold for 5 seconds, breathing normally.
4. Slowly return to the starting position, then repeat.
5. Perform 6 to 8 repetitions on each side.

Alignment Cues
- Keep the cervical spine neutral.
- Align the body before lifting the hips to reduce the risk of back discomfort.
- Lift up out of the bottom shoulder for support.
- Engage the inner thighs to activate the obliques.
- Keep your gaze forward.

Variation
Lift the top hand off the mat and reach upward.

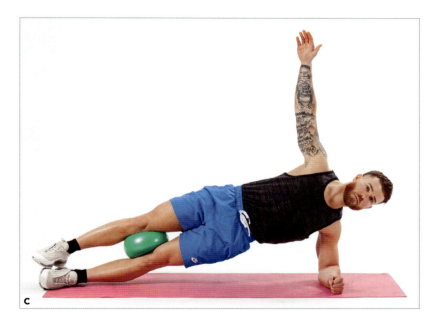
c

One-Handed Side Plank (Ball Between Thighs)

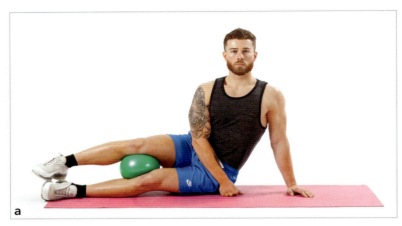

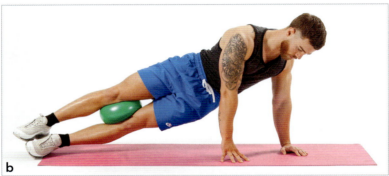

Benefits
The ball assists in engaging the adductors and deep core muscles.

Instructions
1. Begin by sitting on the left side with the hips and knees straight and the ball between the thighs.
2. Place the left hand under the shoulder and the right hand slightly in front of the body to assist in lifting the hips.
3. Lift the left hip off of the floor and hold for 5 seconds, breathing normally.
4. Return the hip to the floor, then repeat.
5. Engage the inner thighs for greater core activation.
6. Perform 6 to 8 repetitions on each side.

Alignment Cues
- Keep the cervical spine neutral.
- Align the body before lifting the hips to reduce the risk of back discomfort.
- Lift up out of the shoulders and the wrists.
- Engage the inner thighs to activate the obliques.
- Keep your gaze forward.

Variation
Take the top hand off of the floor and raise it above the head in a straight line for a greater core challenge.

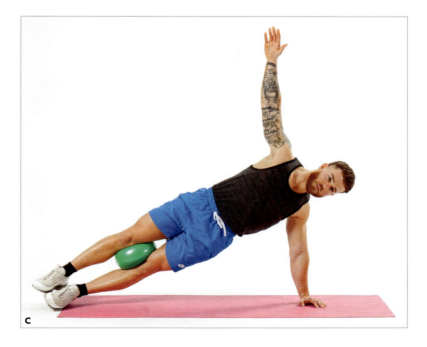
c

Side-Lying Hip Abduction (Ball Under Head)

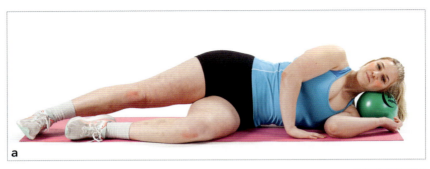

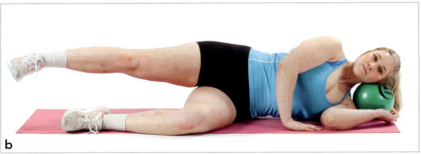

Benefits
The ball helps to stabilize the cervical spine and engage the core while abducting the hip.

Instructions
1. Begin by lying on the left side with the arms in a comfortable position in front of the body.
2. Flex the left hip in front of the body for support.
3. Place the ball under the side of the head (like a pillow).
4. Inhale to initiate.
5. Exhale and abduct the right thigh until it is slightly higher than the right hip.
6. Inhale to return to the starting position, then repeat.
7. Perform 6 to 8 repetitions on each side.

Alignment Cues
- Keep the cervical spine in a neutral position.
- Think of lifting the ribs off the floor to engage the core obliques.
- Abduct the hip only until the gluteus is engaged.
- Move slowly with control.
- Keep your gaze forward.

Side-Lying Hip Abduction (Ball Under Side)

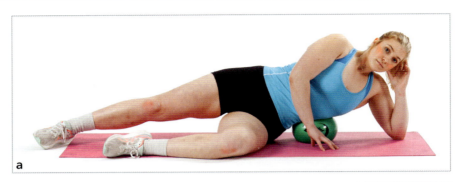

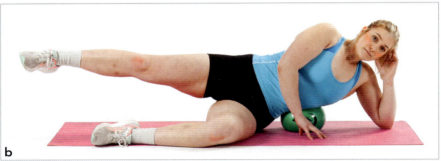

Benefits
The ball helps to activate the sides of the core while protecting the back.

Instructions
1. Begin by lying on the left side with the upper body supported with the ball in between the ribs and the hip.
2. Support the head with the left hand.
3. Keep the right leg straight and the left hip flexed in front of the body for support.
4. Inhale to initiate.
5. Exhale and abduct the right thigh until it is even with the right hip.
6. Moving fluidly, return to the starting position, then repeat on the other side.
7. Perform 6 to 8 repetitions on each side.

Alignment Cues
- Keep the cervical spine neutral.
- Make sure to lift the ribs so as not to collapse into the ball or shoulder.
- Lift the hip only until you feel the glutes engage.
- Move with control.
- Keep your gaze forward.

Variation
Take the supporting elbow off of the floor for a greater core challenge.

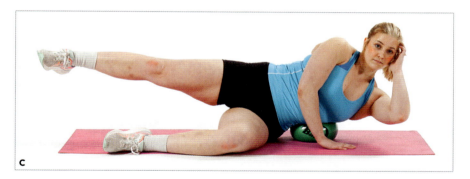

c

Side-Lying Hip Abduction and Lateral Flexion (Ball Under Side)

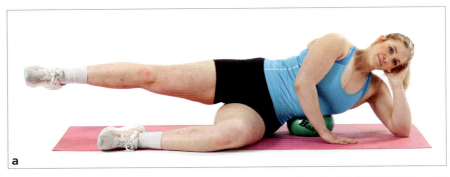

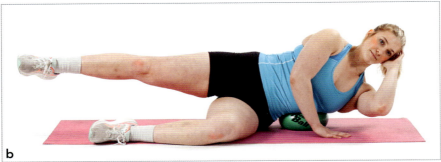

Benefits
The ball supports the core during lateral flexion of the spine while abducting the hip.

Instructions
1. Begin by lying on the left side with the left hand supporting the head and the ball in between the ribs and the hip.
2. The right leg is straight and the right hand is in front of the body for support.
3. The left hip and knee are flexed in front of the body.
4. Inhale to initiate.
5. Exhale, abducting the right thigh and laterally flexing the torso at the same time.
6. Moving fluidly, inhale to return to the starting position, then repeat.
7. Perform 6 to 8 repetitions on each side.

Alignment Cues
- Keep the cervical spine neutral.
- Lift the torso only until the obliques are engaged.
- Abduct the hip only until the glutes are engaged.
- Move with control.
- Keep your gaze forward.

110 Vital Core Training

Side-Lying Hip Abduction and Lateral Flexion With Glider Disc (Ball Under Side)

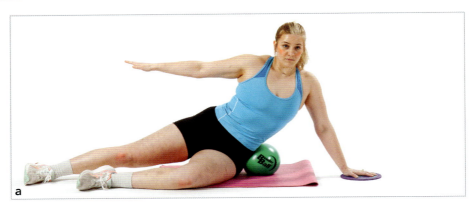
a

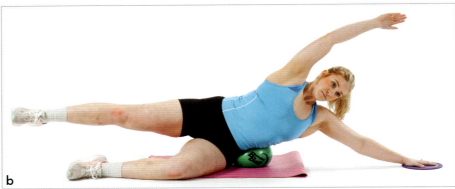
b

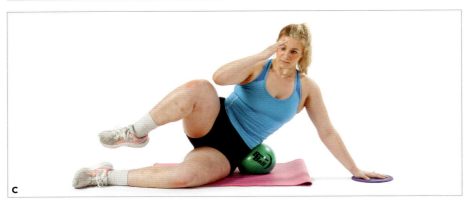
c

Benefits
The ball and glider disc combine to support the core when laterally flexing. If a glider disc is not available, you can also use another implement such as a towel or paper plate.

Instructions
1. Begin by sitting on the mat with the ball securely placed next to the left hip.
2. Place the left hand on the glider disc with the shoulder at a slight angle in front of the body.
3. The right arm is to the side of the body, and the right hip and knee are straight.
4. Flex the left knee and hip in front of the body for support.
5. Inhale to initiate, extending the right arm over the head and abducting the right hip.
6. Exhale and while moving fluidly, flex the spine and hip toward the midline of the body.
7. Perform 6 to 8 repetitions on each side.

Alignment Cues
- Make sure to slide the hand away and return with control.
- Lift the torso only until the obliques are engaged.
- Abduct the hip only until the outer thighs are engaged.
- Keep your gaze forward.

CHAPTER 7

Seated and Supine Exercises

Positioning the small ball behind the low back can offer additional support, strength, and functionality while performing the exercises described in this chapter, which is vital for injury prevention and integrity of the spine. Many people place their bodies into hip flexion by sitting for long periods or performing supine crunches for core exercise, but these positions may cause the muscles in the front of the body, especially the rectus abdominis and hip flexors, to become short, tight, and weak and place undue stress on the low back. The ball helps create extension and load on these muscles, which is otherwise difficult to achieve in a seated or supine position. It does not take many repetitions of seated and supine exercises with the small ball to feel the intensity, even for the strongest core enthusiast.

The exercises and stretches are color coded. Exercises in green are for all levels of participants. Exercises in blue are slightly more challenging yet appropriate for most participants. Exercises in red are for higher-level participants looking for a more challenging exercise.

You will find that most of the exercises in this text are suitable for everyone. However, if an exercise seems too difficult, then alignment or outcome can be compromised; therefore, make sure the exercise feels good to the client's body so the goal can be achieved. Keep in mind that good alignment and form are more important than anything else with all exercises in this program.

Benefits and Cues

Using the ball with seated and supine exercises provides several benefits. The small ball can

- help align the back and hips,
- protect and provide a more comfortable position for the low and mid back,
- allow for deeper core activation, and
- offer more intense and effective execution of the exercises.

The following alignment cues should be reviewed before undertaking the exercises:

- When using the ball behind the low back, wedge the ball securely; you should feel the support slightly above the tailbone (a).
- When using the ball behind the shoulder blades, make sure to support the head with the hands (b).
- Do not extend to the point of discomfort when executing any exercise.
- Always move within the appropriate range of motion (until you feel the muscles in the front of the body engage).
- Keep the feet on the floor or the glider disc to keep the focus on the anterior core muscles rather than the hip flexors (c).

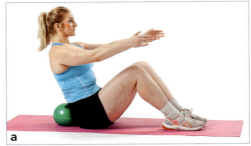

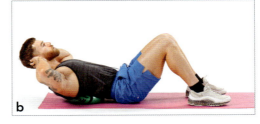

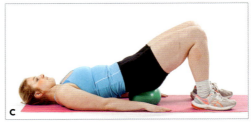

SEATED EXERCISES

Seated Anterior Core Lengthening (Ball Behind Mid Back)

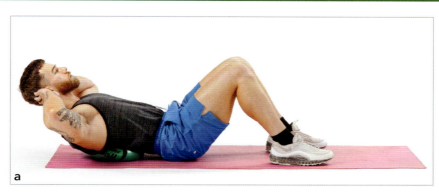

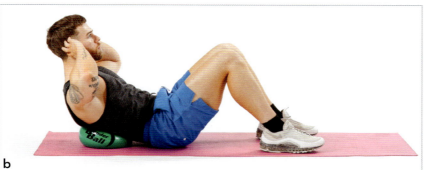

Benefits
The ball allows the thoracic spine to extend while supporting the head.

Instructions
1. Begin seated in a reclined position with the hips on the mat and the ball behind the mid back in between the shoulder blades.
2. Keep the knees bent and the feet on the mat.
3. Support the head with the hands and the elbows extended so you can see them in your peripheral vision.
4. Inhale to initiate, extending the thoracic spine slightly.
5. Exhale to slightly flex the spine.
6. Moving fluidly, return to the starting position.
7. Perform 6 to 8 repetitions.

Alignment Cues
- Keep the spine neutral to begin and slightly extended during the movement.
- Keep your gaze forward.
- Do not hyperextend the spine over the ball, creating discomfort.
- Keep the head supported at all times.

Seated Anterior Core Lengthening (Ball Behind Low Back)

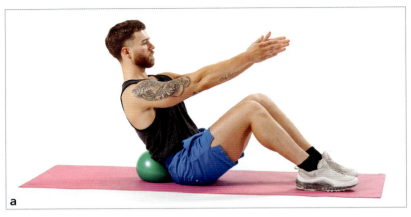

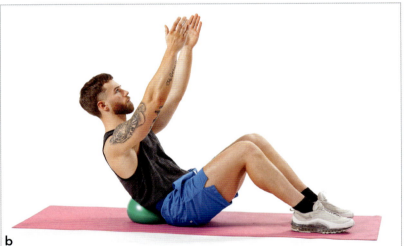

Benefits
Placing the ball behind the low back provides support and allows the front of the body to lengthen and engage against gravity.

Instructions
1. Sitting with the knees and hips flexed and the feet on the floor, place the ball securely behind the low back and reach the arms in front of the chest. The lumbar spine should be slightly curved and the hips should be relaxed.
2. Inhale to initiate.
3. Moving fluidly, exhale slightly and lean back. Reach the arms upward until the core engages.
4. Perform 6 to 8 repetitions.

Alignment Cues
- Keep the cervical spine neutral and the thoracic spine extended.
- Lean back only until the front of the body is engaged.
- Move slowly.
- Keep your gaze slightly upward.

Variation
You can increase the intensity of the exercise by abducting the arms to the sides and holding weights.

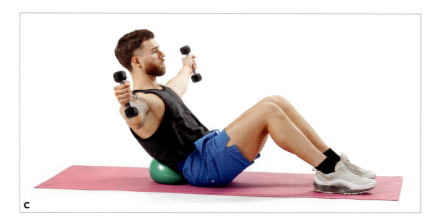

SAFETY TIP If additional support is needed, place the hand on the outer thigh for balance.

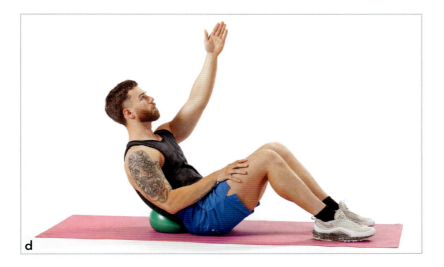

Seated Anterior Core Lengthening With Chair

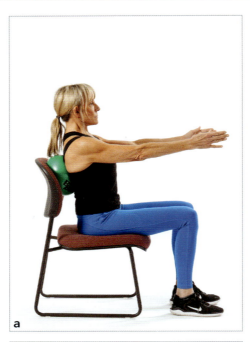

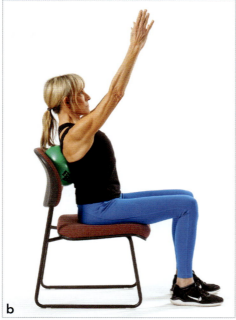

Seated and Supine Exercises 119

Benefits
For an individual who cannot get up and down from the floor or for someone sitting at a desk, using a chair with back support is a good option.

Instructions
1. Sitting upright with good posture in a supported chair, place the ball securely behind the mid to upper back.
2. Make sure the feet are placed on the floor and the arms are extended in front of the chest.
3. Press the back into the chair to feel the core engage.
4. Inhale to initiate.
5. Exhale, reaching the arms upward.
6. Perform 6 to 8 repetitions.

Alignment Cues
- Keep the cervical spine neutral.
- Lean back only until the front of the body is engaged.
- Move slowly.
- Keep your gaze slightly upward.

Variation
Abduct the arms to the sides of the body.

SAFETY TIP If additional support is needed, place the hands on the thighs for balance.

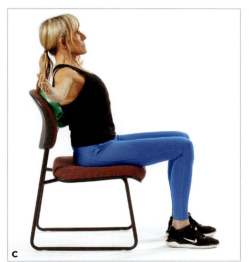
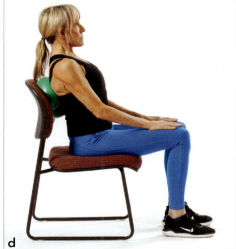

Seated Anterior Core Lengthening With Glider Disc (Ball Behind Low Back)

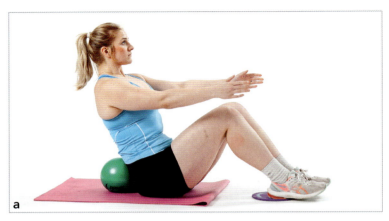

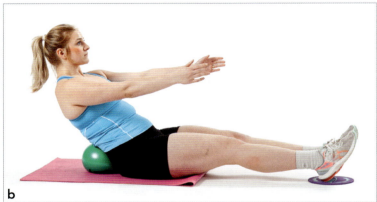

Benefits
Using a glider disc to extend the legs engages the core muscles even further and allows for more lengthening. If a glider disc is not available, you can also use another implement such as a towel or paper plate.

Instructions
1. Sit upright with the ball securely wedged behind the low back.
2. Place the heels on the glider disc with the knees bent and the arms in front of the body.
3. Inhale to initiate.
4. Exhale, pressing the low back into the ball, reaching the arms up, and straightening the knees.
5. Moving fluidly, return to the starting position.
6. Perform 6 to 8 repetitions.

Seated and Supine Exercises 121

Alignment Cues
- Keep the cervical spine neutral.
- Lean back only until the anterior core is engaged.
- Move slowly.
- Keep the feet on the glider disc throughout the movement.
- Keep your gaze upward.

Variations
To make the exercise more intense, raise the arms over the shoulders. To add more challenge, hold a weight in each hand throughout the movement.

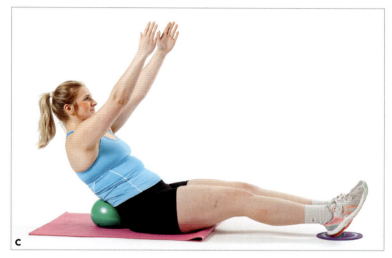

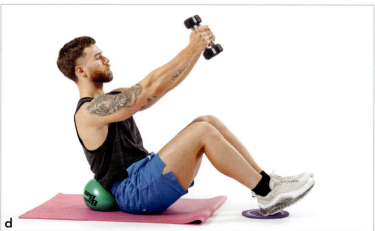

Seated Anterior and Lateral Core Rotation (Ball Behind Low Back)

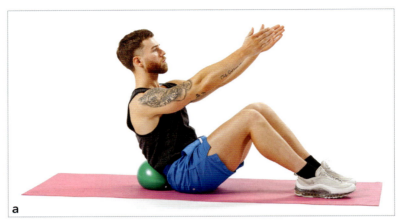

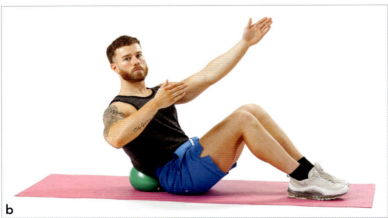

Benefits
Placing the ball behind the low back provides support and allows the front and side of the body to lengthen and engage against gravity. The rotation is more functional than performing supine crunches.

Instructions
1. Sit upright with the ball securely wedged behind the low back (sacrum) and the knees bent.
2. Inhale to initiate, extending the arms in front of the body.
3. Exhale, slowly rotating to the right. Bend the right elbow while keeping the right arm at the side.
4. Gaze over the right shoulder while extending the left arm slightly to the side and above the shoulder.
5. Moving fluidly, return to the starting position and repeat on the left side.
6. Perform 6 to 8 repetitions on each side.

Alignment Cues
- Rotate only until the elbow is either to the side of the shoulder or just above the mat.
- Move slowly into the rotation.
- Keep the feet on the mat.
- Focus on the side body when rotating to engage the core.
- Keep your gaze in the direction of rotation.

Variation
For added challenge, lower the right elbow and open the chest by reaching and opening the left arm out to the side of the body.

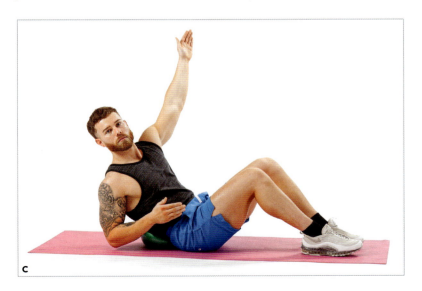

c

Seated Anterior and Lateral Core Rotation With Glider Disc (Ball Behind Low Back)

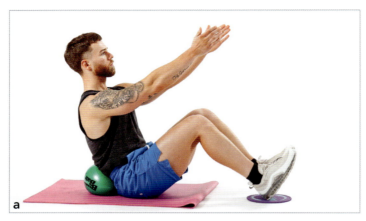

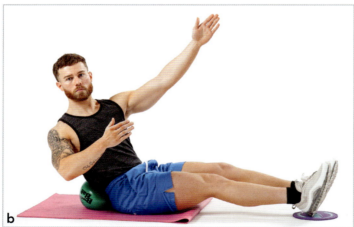

Benefits

Placing the ball behind the low back provides support and allows the front and side of the body to lengthen against gravity. Using a glider disc increases the intensity by also engaging the lower body. If a glider disc is not available, you can also use another implement such as a towel or paper plate.

Instructions

1. Sitting with good posture, securely place the ball behind the low back. The lumbar spine should be slightly curved.
2. Place the heels on the glider disc and raise the arms in front of the body.
3. Inhale to initiate.
4. Exhale, extending the knees and hips while rotating the spine to the right.
5. Gaze in the direction of the torso while keeping the right elbow bent and to the side of the shoulder.
6. Extend the left arm slightly to the side and above the shoulder.
7. Return to the starting position and repeat on the left.
8. Perform 6 to 8 repetitions on each side.

Alignment Cues

- Do not lean back too far.
- Move slowly.
- Keep a slight bend in the knees while extending the hips.
- Think of pulling the legs back to the body with the core and not the hip flexors.
- Rotate the spine only until you feel the front and side of the body engage.
- Keep your gaze in the direction of rotation.

Variations

To make the exercise more challenging, reach one arm above the shoulder. For more intensity, hold a weight in each hand throughout the movement.

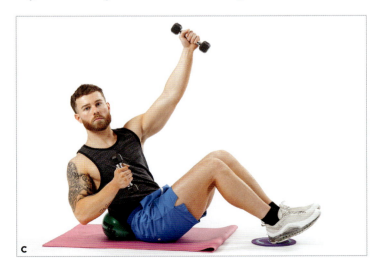

Seated Anterior and Lateral Core Lengthening (Ball Behind Mid Back)

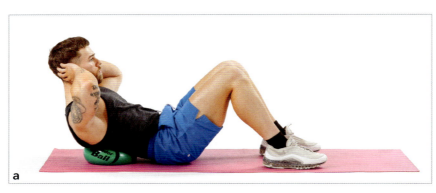

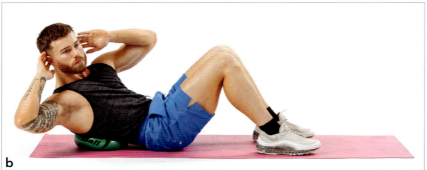

Benefits
Placing the ball behind the mid back provides elevation off the floor to allow the thoracic spine to extend and laterally flex, which otherwise cannot be achieved.

Instructions
1. Begin seated in a reclined position with the hips on the mat and the ball behind the mid back in between the shoulder blades.
2. Keep the knees bent and the feet on the mat.
3. Support the head with the hands and the elbows extended so you can see them in your peripheral vision.
4. Inhale to initiate, extending the thoracic spine slightly.
5. Exhale to slightly flex and rotate the spine to the right.
6. Moving fluidly, return to the starting position.
7. Perform 6 to 8 repetitions on each side.

Alignment Cues
- Keep the spine neutral to begin and slightly extended during the movement.
- Do not hyperextend the spine over the ball, creating discomfort.
- Keep the head supported at all times.

Seated and Supine Exercises   127

SUPINE EXERCISES

Bridge (Ball Under Sacrum)

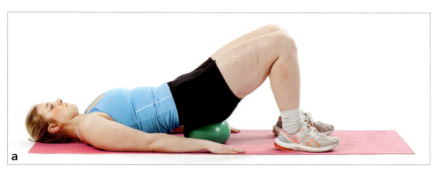

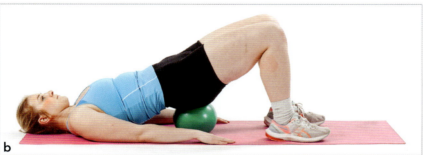

Benefits
Placing the ball under the sacrum provides support and elevation to engage and lengthen the front of the body.

Instructions
1. Lying on the back on the mat with the knees bent and the arms on the floor alongside the body, place the ball directly under the sacrum.
2. Position the knees approximately hip-width apart.
3. Press the palms into the mat so the arms are an active part of the exercise.
4. Let the ball support the body.
5. Inhale to initiate, lifting the sacrum slightly off the ball in a neutral spine.
6. Hold for 5 seconds, breathing normally.
7. Lower the sacrum until you feel the support of the ball.
8. Perform 6 to 8 repetitions.

Alignment Cues
- Do not hyperextend the low back.
- Do not squeeze, tighten, or tuck the glutes or pelvis, which will restrict movement.
- Keep the spine neutral.
- Think of lengthening the front of the body.

Bridge (Ball Between Knees)

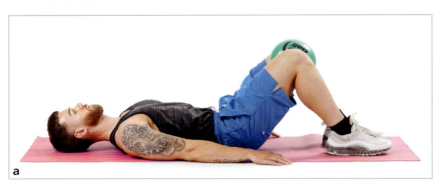

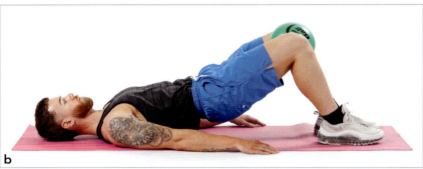

Benefits
Placing the ball between the knees allows for deeper and more efficient muscle activation of the pelvic floor muscles. It also helps align and stabilize the hips.

Instructions
1. Lying on the back with the knees bent and the arms on the mat alongside the body, place the ball between the thighs just above the knees.
2. Position the feet hip-width apart or slightly narrower to keep the ball in place.
3. Press the palms into the mat so the arms are an active part of the exercise.
4. Inhale to initiate.
5. Exhale and lift the hips into a neutral bridge, engaging the inner thighs.
6. Hold for 5 seconds, breathing normally.
7. Lower the hips to the starting position.
8. Perform 6 to 8 repetitions.

Alignment Cues
- Do not hyperextend the low back.
- Keep the spine neutral.
- Do not squeeze, tighten, or tuck the glutes or pelvis, which will restrict movement.
- Think of lifting the hips with the least amount of effort possible to lengthen the front of the body.
- Keep a slight engagement of the inner thighs throughout the movement.

Variation
Deepen your body awareness by alternating pressure on the ball with the thighs. While lifting the hips into a bridge, focus on lengthening the front of the body and right inner thigh. Alternate engaging the right and left thigh with each lift of the hips.

Bridge (Ball Under Foot)

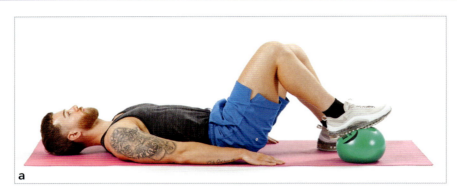

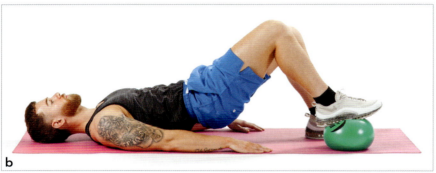

Benefits
Placing the ball under one foot creates instability and greater engagement of the core.

Instructions
1. Lie on the back with the knees bent and the feet positioned hip-width apart. Place the arms on the mat alongside the body.
2. Place the ball under the arch of the right foot.
3. Position the left foot in line with the left hip to assist with balance.
4. Inhale to initiate.
5. Exhale, lifting the hips to a neutral position, focusing on the right side of the body.
6. Press the arch of the right foot slightly into the ball.
7. Hold for 5 seconds, breathing normally.
8. Lower the hips to the starting position.
9. Perform 6 to 8 repetitions on each side, either by alternating to give the hamstrings a rest or performing all repetitions on one side before switching to the other.

Alignment Cues
- Keep the spine neutral.
- Do not hyperextend the low back.
- Do not squeeze, tighten, or tuck the glutes or pelvis, which will restrict movement.
- Engage the side of the body on the same side as the ball.
- Focus on lengthening the front of the body.

Bridge (Ball on Thighs)

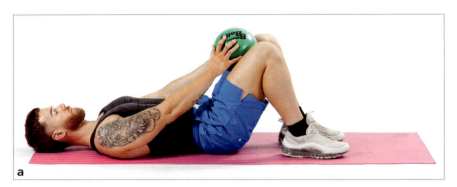

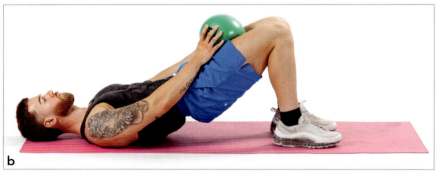

Benefits
Pressing into the ball on the thighs activates the deeper core muscles and increases intra-abdominal pressure.

Instructions
1. Lie on the back on the mat with the knees bent. Position the hips and knees close together enough to place the ball on top of the thighs.
2. Place both hands on the ball and apply pressure.
3. Inhale to initiate.
4. Exhale, lifting the hips to a neutral position and pressing the hands into the ball until activation of the core is felt.
5. Hold for 5 seconds, breathing normally.
6. Lower the hips to the starting position.
7. Perform 6 to 8 repetitions.

Alignment Cues
- Keep the spine neutral.
- Do not hyperextend the low back.
- Do not squeeze, tighten, or tuck the glutes, which will restrict movement.
- Apply only slight pressure with the hands.

Bridge With Hip Flexion (Ball on Thigh)

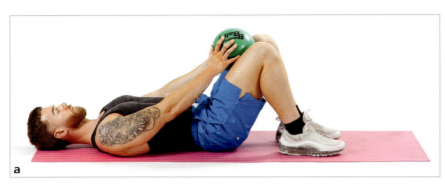

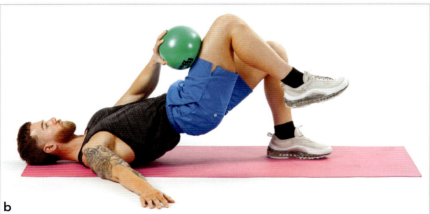

Benefits
Pressing into the ball on one thigh creates instability and activates the core more efficiently.

Instructions
1. Lie on the back on the mat with the knees bent. Position the hips and knees close together enough to place the ball on top of the thighs.
2. Place the right arm next to the body, holding the ball against the right thigh with the left hand.
3. Inhale to initiate.
4. Exhale, lifting the hips to a neutral position and hover the right foot off the floor while gently pressing the hand into the ball.
5. Hold for 5 seconds, breathing normally.
6. Lower to the starting position.
7. Perform 6 to 8 repetitions on each side, either by alternating to give the hamstrings a rest or performing all repetitions on one side before switching to the other.

Alignment Cues
- Keep the spine neutral.
- Do not hyperextend the low back.
- Do not squeeze, tighten, or tuck the glutes or pelvis, which will restrict movement.
- Press into the ball only hard enough to activate the core.

Toe Taps (Ball Under Sacrum)

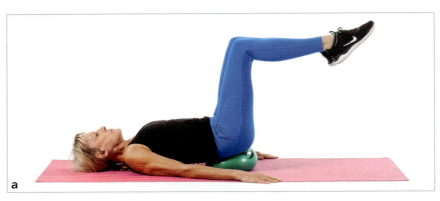

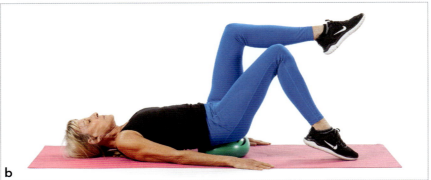

Benefits
Placing the ball under the sacrum creates a stability challenge while protecting the low back.

Instructions
1. Lie on the back on the mat and place the ball under the sacrum.
2. Bend the knees to 90 degrees.
3. Place the arms on the mat alongside the body.
4. Inhale to initiate.
5. Exhale, slowly lowering the right leg to tap the right toes to the floor.
6. Slowly bring the right leg back to 90 degrees, then repeat on the other side.
7. Perform 6 to 8 repetitions on each side.

Alignment Cues
- Keep the hips stable and flexed at 90 degrees so that you do not overuse the hip flexors.
- Focus on maintaining stability in the core as you move the legs.

Variation
To add challenge, reach the arms toward the ceiling in the starting position. While lowering the right leg to tap the toes to the floor, extend the left arm overhead at the same time. Inhale to bring the leg and arm back to the start, then alternate on the next repetition (left leg and right arm move). Move slowly and intentionally while concentrating on keeping the body as still as possible, which will activate the core.

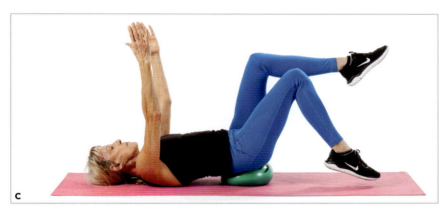

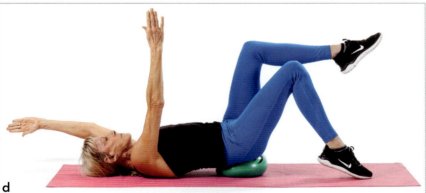

Hip and Knee Extension (Ball Under Sacrum)

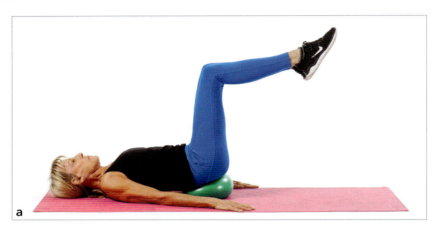

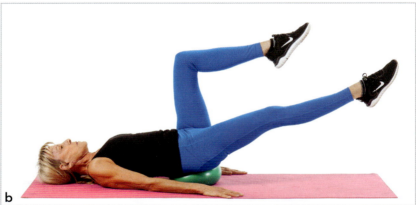

Benefits
Placing the ball under the sacrum and alternating hip extensions provides a greater challenge for hamstring flexibility and core activation.

Instructions
1. Lie on the back on the mat and place the ball under the sacrum.
2. Bend the knees to 90 degrees.
3. Place the arms on the mat alongside the body.
4. Inhale to initiate.
5. Exhale, slowly extending the right knee and hip, keeping the left knee bent.
6. Slowly bring the right leg back to the starting position, then repeat on the other side.
7. Perform 6 to 8 repetitions on each side.

Alignment Cues
- Keep the legs within 90- to 45-degree angles to protect the low back.
- Move slowly and with control throughout the movement, focusing on maintaining stability.
- Think of lengthening the hip flexors when lowering each leg.

Variation
For an additional challenge, hover the hands and arms above the chest. This movement creates instability that further engages the core.

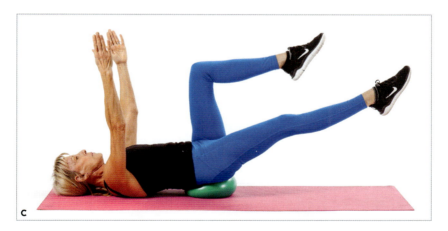

Hip Flexion (Ball on Thigh)

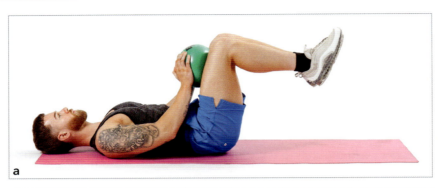

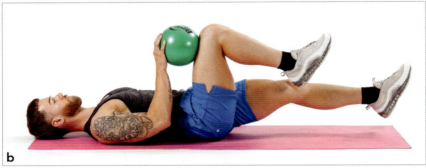

Benefits
This exercise engages the deep core muscles while keeping the spine neutral.

Instructions
1. Lie on the back on the mat with a neutral spine.
2. Bend the knees to 90 degrees.
3. Place the ball on the right thigh while pressing it with both hands.
4. Inhale to initiate.
5. Exhale, extending the left thigh and knee slightly above the mat.
6. Return to the starting position.
7. Perform 6 to 8 repetitions on each side, either by alternating or performing all repetitions on one side before switching to the other.

Alignment Cues
- Keep the spine neutral.
- Make sure to return the hips to 90 degrees at the end of each repetition.
- Move slowly and with control throughout the movement, focusing on stabilizing the hips.
- Focus on the lifting and lowering of the leg while pressing the ball gently into the other leg.

Variation
For a regression, keep the left arm along the left side, palm facing downward. This position can assist with balance.

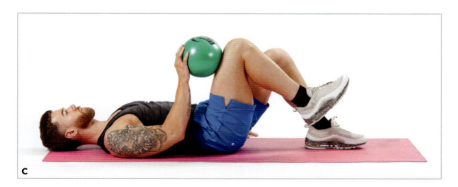

c

SAFETY TIP If there is discomfort, you may keep the knees flexed instead of extended.

Hip Flexion With Toe Taps (Ball on Thighs)

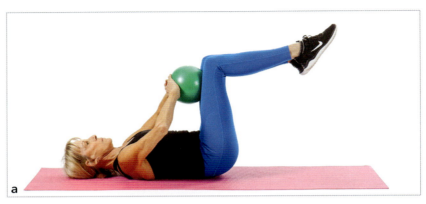

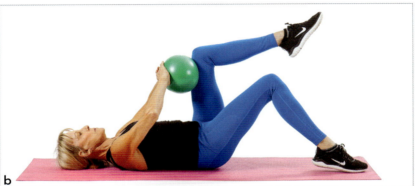

Benefits
This exercise engages the deep core muscles while keeping the hips stable.

Instructions
1. Lie on the back on the mat with a neutral spine, keeping the knees together.
2. Bend the knees to 90 degrees.
3. Place the ball on both thighs, pressing the hands into the ball.
4. Inhale to initiate.
5. Exhale, slowly tapping the right toes to the mat.
6. Keep the pelvis still during the movement.
7. Perform 6 to 8 repetitions on each side, alternating right and left.

Alignment Cues
- Keep the spine neutral.
- Keep the hips stable.
- Move slowly and with control, focusing on alternating the toe taps to activate the deep core muscles.

Variation
Extend the right hip and knee for deeper core activation.

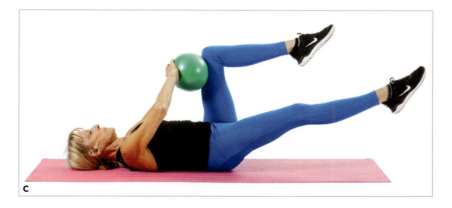
c

CHAPTER 8

Stretches

This chapter focuses on lengthening and stretching the body's core using the ball for support, which promotes relaxation and improves mobility and suppleness. Pairing relaxation with breath work will promote better health and longevity. When your exercise routine includes stretching and relaxation, it stimulates recovery.

It is vital to have the ball placed in the correct position in order for the exercises to be safe and effective. Move only to the point of feeling the desired outcome of the stretching.

The exercises and stretches are color coded. Exercises in green are for all levels of participants. Exercises in blue are slightly more challenging yet appropriate for most participants. Exercises in red are for higher-level participants looking for a more challenging exercise.

You will find that most of the exercises in this text are suitable for everyone. However, if an exercise seems too difficult, then alignment or outcome can be compromised; therefore, make sure the exercise feels good to the client's body so the goal can be achieved. Keep in mind that good alignment and form are more important than anything else with all exercises in this program.

Benefits and Cues

Using the ball correctly with stretches provides several benefits. The small ball can

- increase range of motion,
- provide kinesthetic feedback, and
- provide support for the low back and hips.

The following alignment cues should be reviewed before undertaking the exercises:

- Never hyperextend the spine *(a)*.
- Never stretch to the point of pain—stretching should feel good.
- Keep the spine neutral as much as possible *(b)*.

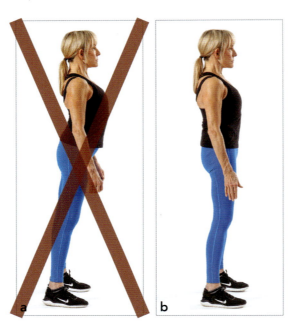

Learn to Breathe

The body is much more responsive when you allow yourself to let go of emotions while stretching. Inhaling deeply through the nose and exhaling slowly through the mouth or nose has a calming effect on the nervous system. Stretches will be easier to achieve when you breathe deeply and focus on relaxing and releasing negative thoughts. Simply breathe in and out when holding your stretch, trying not to hold your breath.

Gentle Stretching

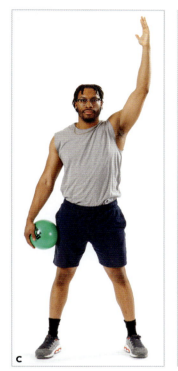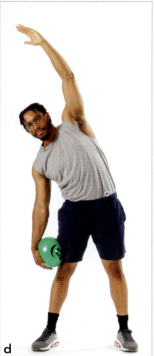

When a muscle is stretched beyond comfort, it will potentially contract in response as a protective mechanism, which is called the *stretch reflex*. Therefore, a gentle stretch—rather than pulsing or forcing—is best to allow the tissue to respond and lengthen *(c, d)*. Gentle stretching is simply applying a little resistance on an area of the body and then releasing it. This can be performed as slowly as needed on each side of the body.

Holding a Stretch

When holding a stretch, focus on the area of the body that the stretch is designed to target. If there are any restrictions, limit the range of motion to avoid causing pain or discomfort. A good benchmark for holding a stretch is 10 seconds; longer is better because the muscle will have a tendency to relax.

Side Bend

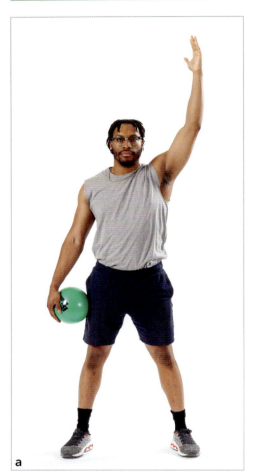
a

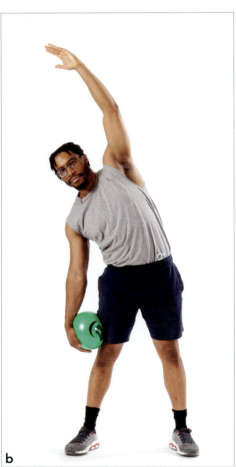
b

Benefits
This stretch lengthens the lateral side of the body, specifically the hips, for increased mobility.

Instructions
1. Standing with the feet slightly wider than hip-width apart and the knees soft, hold the ball against the right hip with the right hand.
2. Inhale to initiate.
3. Exhale, pressing the ball into the hip, extending the left arm overhead, and laterally flexing to the right.
4. Hold for 5 to 10 seconds, breathing normally.
5. Return to the starting position, then repeat.
6. Perform as needed on each side, completing the repetitions on one side of the body before switching sides.

Alignment Cues
- Make sure not to pulse, but gently stretch into the hip.
- Focus on lengthening the side of the body.

Side Bend With Legs Crossed

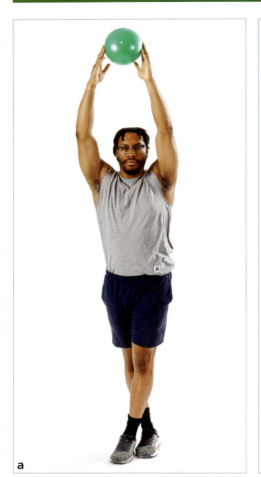
a

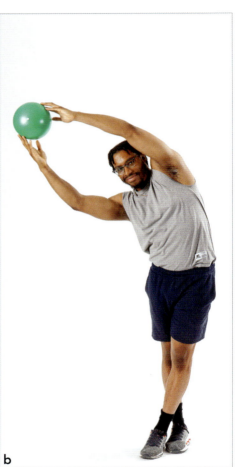
b

Benefits
This stretch lengthens the lateral side of the body, specifically the hips, for increased mobility. Crossing one leg over the other creates more of an immediate stretch in the lateral hip.

Instructions
1. Standing with the left leg crossed over the right, hold the ball overhead.
2. Inhale to initiate.
3. Exhale, pressing the left hand into the ball while laterally flexing the spine to the right.
4. Hold for 5 to 10 seconds, breathing normally.
5. Return to the starting position, then repeat.
6. Perform as needed on each side, completing the repetitions on one side of the body before crossing the right leg over the left to switch sides.

Alignment Cues
- Make sure not to pulse, but gently stretch into the hip.
- Focus on lengthening the side of the body.

152 Vital Core Training

Posterior Cross Lunge

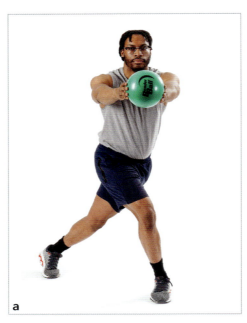
a

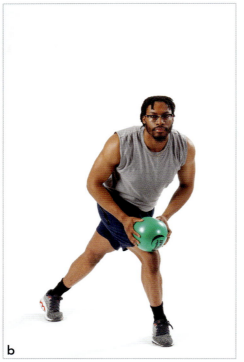
b

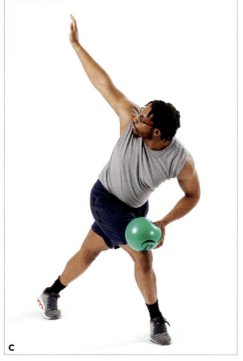
c

Benefits
This stretch lengthens the posterior body, specifically the hip complex.

Instructions
1. Begin by standing with the left leg crossed behind the right, arms in front of the body and holding the ball in both hands.
2. Hinge forward until the right glute and hamstring engage, then press the ball against the right thigh slightly more with the left hand.
3. Inhale to initiate.
4. Exhale, slowly rotating the thoracic spine to the right and extending the right arm toward the ceiling.
5. Hold the stretch 5 to 10 seconds, breathing normally.
6. Return to the starting position, then repeat.
7. Perform as needed on each side, completing the repetitions on one side of the body before switching sides.

Alignment Cues
- Rotate only until you feel a stretch in the obliques and hips.
- Stay within your range of motion.

Inner Thigh Stretch

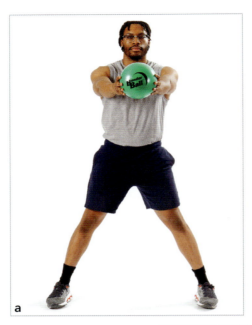

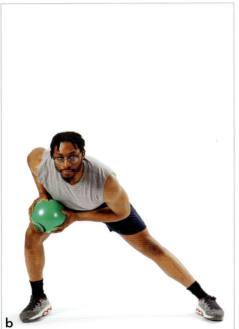
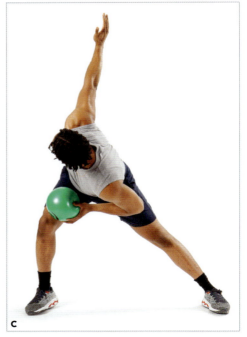

Benefits
This stretch enhances flexibility and mobility of the hips and the adductors.

Instructions
1. Standing with the feet more than hip-width apart and the knees soft, hold the ball with both hands in front of the body.
2. Inhale to initiate.
3. Exhale, flexing the right knee to come into a side-lunge position.
4. Place the ball on the top of the right thigh pressing slightly more with the left hand and rotate the thoracic spine to the right.
5. Raise the right arm above the body, palm facing outward, to align with the right leg.
6. Keep the left knee extended and focus on lengthening the left adductor.
7. Hold for 5 to 10 seconds, breathing normally.
8. Return to the starting position, then repeat.
9. Perform as needed on each side, completing the repetitions on one side of the body before switching sides.

Alignment Cues
- Make sure to place the ball where you need it to feel the stretch.
- Move slowly so as not to overstretch the adductors.
- Flex the knee only until you feel a stretch in the opposite adductor.
- Stay within your range of motion.
- Make sure the feet are parallel or slightly externally rotated.

Vertical Rotation

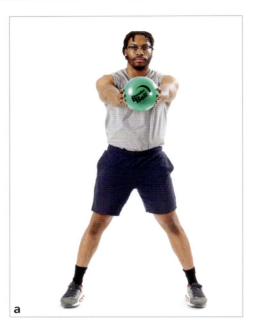

a

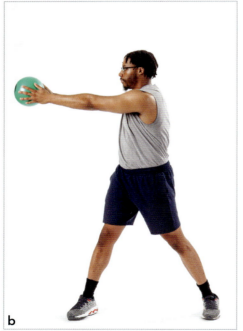

b

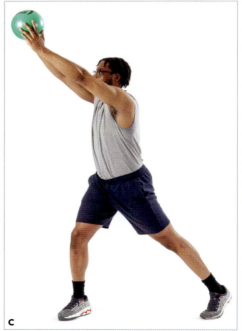

c

Benefits
This stretch lengthens the side body and is great for those who participate in rotational sports such as golf or tennis.

Instructions
1. Standing with the feet slightly wider than hip-width apart and the arms extended in front of you at shoulder height, hold the ball in both hands.
2. Inhale to initiate.
3. Exhale, rotating the thoracic spine to the right, keeping the arms at chest height.
4. While you are still rotated to the right, reach the arms over the shoulders, pressing into the ball slightly more with the left hand.
5. Hold for 5 to 10 seconds, breathing normally.
6. Return to the starting position, then repeat on the other side.
7. Perform as needed on each side.

Alignment Cues
- Let the hips rotate with the thoracic spine.
- Imagine lifting out of the hips, creating space and growing taller as you rotate and extend the arms.

Thread the Needle

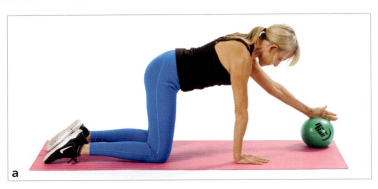

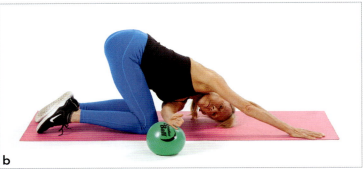

Benefits
The ball offers assistance and elevation for those with tight shoulders.

Instructions
1. Kneeling on the hands and knees in a tabletop position on a mat, place the ball on the ground underneath the left hand, with the thumb facing up.
2. Inhale to initiate.
3. Exhale, rotating the thoracic spine to the right and rolling the ball under the body.
4. Keep the hips lifted.
5. Hold for 5 to 10 seconds, breathing normally.
6. Perform as needed on each side, completing the repetitions on one side of the body before switching sides.

Alignment Cues
- Move slowly and without shoulder impingement.
- Keep to a small range of motion, gently rocking back and forth.
- Positioning the thumb pointing up provides slight internal rotation for the shoulder. You can always adjust the position of the hand depending on flexibility.

Pectoralis Stretch

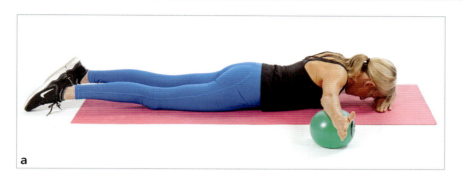

Benefits
Placing the ball under the hand elevates the shoulder for a deeper stretch and allows the chest to open.

Instructions
1. Lie prone on a mat with the forehead resting on the left forearm and the right arm abducted to the side of the body.
2. Place the ball under the right forearm or hand.
3. Inhale to initiate.
4. Exhale, gently pressing into the ball.
5. Hold for 5 to 10 seconds, breathing normally.
6. Perform as needed on each side, completing the repetitions on one side of the body before switching sides.

Alignment Cues
- Move slowly and without shoulder impingement or discomfort.
- Keep within a small range of motion.
- Always support the head and neck with the opposite forearm.

Variation
Bend the elbow to decrease the intensity of the stretch.

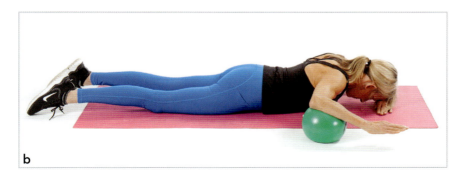

Side-Lying Stretch

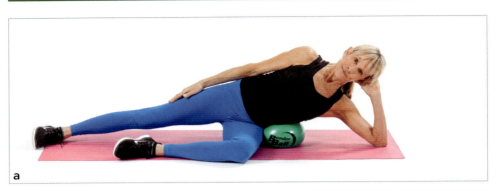

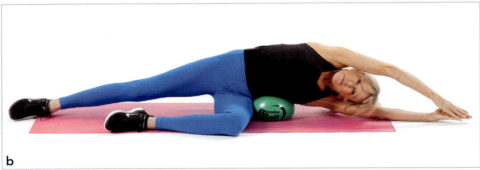

Benefits
Placing the ball under the rib cage allows for a deeper lateral stretch of the core.

Instructions
1. Begin by lying on the left side on a mat with the left hand supporting the head, the right leg straight, the left hip flexed in front of the body for support, and the ball under the rib cage and hip.
2. Inhale to initiate.
3. Exhale to reach the right arm over the shoulder to gently stretch the right side of the body, then extend the left arm so both are overhead.
4. Hold for 5 to 10 seconds, breathing normally.
5. Return to the starting position, then repeat.
6. Perform as needed on each side, completing the repetitions on one side of the body before switching sides.

Alignment Cues
- Imagine lengthening the side of the body, creating space between the ribs.
- Move slowly and with control.

SAFETY TIPS   Reach the arm only as far as it is comfortable. Do not stretch to any point of discomfort. Always support the head and neck.

Supine Rotation

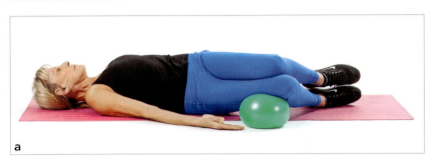
a

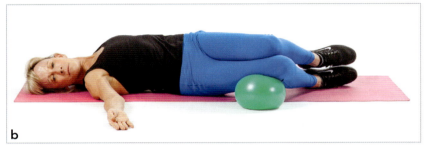
b

Benefits
Placing the ball under the knees provides elevation and easier rotation for those with a tight low back and hips or sensitive knees.

Instructions
1. Lying on the back on a mat with the hips and knees flexed, hold the ball on the mat on the right side of the body using the right hand. The left arm can either be alongside the body or abducted to the side for a deeper stretch.
2. Inhale to initiate.
3. Exhale, rotating the hips to the right so that the right knee rests on top of the ball.
4. Hold for at least 5 to 10 seconds, breathing normally.
5. Return to the starting position, then repeat.
6. Perform as needed on each side, completing the repetitions on one side of the body before switching sides.

Alignment Cues
- Make sure to let the knee rest on the ball.
- Move slowly into the rotation.
- Keep the neck in a comfortable position and turn the head the same direction as the knees for less of a stretch.

Variation
Placing the ball between the knees during this stretch can help activate the adductors. While rotating the legs to one side, allow the top knee to gently press into the ball to engage the adductor muscles.

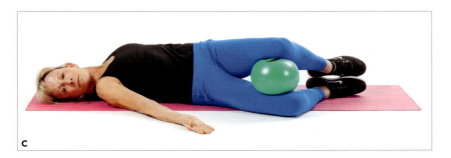

c

Butterfly Stretch

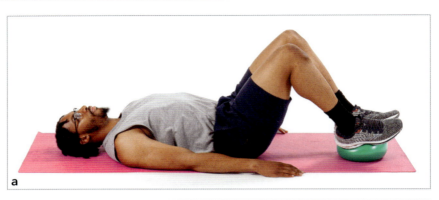

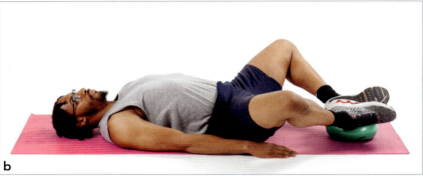

Benefits
Placing the feet on the ball during the stretch provides elevation for those with tight hips.

Instructions
1. Lying on the back on a mat with the knees bent and the arms resting alongside the body, place the arches of both feet on the ball.
2. Inhale to initiate.
3. Exhale and slowly let the knees fall out to either side, allowing the hips to only abduct as far as feels comfortable.
4. Hold for at least 5 to 10 seconds, breathing normally.
5. Return to the starting position and repeat.
6. Perform as needed.

Alignment Cues
- Do not bounce or pulse, which could cause pain in the adductors.
- Move slowly into the stretch.

Hip Flexor Stretch

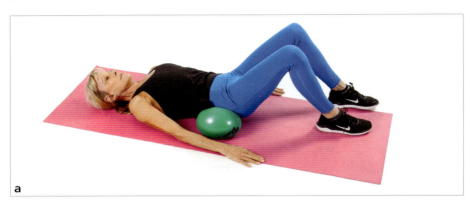

a

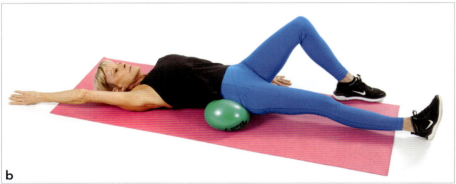

b

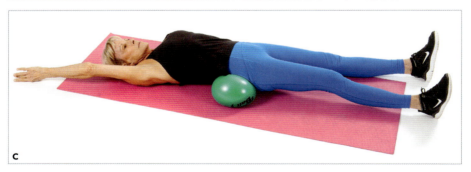

c

Benefits
Placing the ball underneath one buttock allows the hip to be slightly elevated, creating a greater stretch for the hip flexor.

Instructions
1. Lying on the back on a mat with the knees bent and the arms alongside the body, place approximately half of the ball underneath the right buttock only, keeping the left buttock on the mat.
2. Inhale to initiate.
3. Exhale, extending the right arm overhead, followed by extending the right hip and knee. Keep the right heel on the floor.
4. Straighten the left hip and knee, keeping the left heel on the floor.
5. Allow the body to relax, slowly dorsiflexing and plantar flexing the ankles with each breath.
6. Stretch for at least 30 to 60 seconds, breathing normally. The stretch can be held for longer if needed.
7. Perform as needed on each side.

Alignment Cues
- Keep one hip on the floor so the other is elevated.
- Make sure only part of the ball is under the hip, not the entire ball.
- Think of lengthening and creating space between the ribs and the hip.

Hamstring Stretch

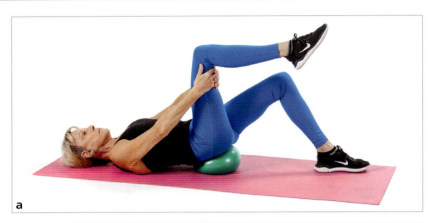

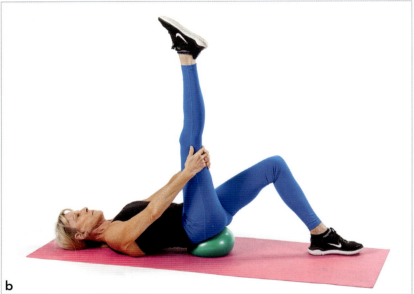

Benefits
Placing the ball under the sacrum elevates the hips, which can be beneficial for anyone with tight hamstrings.

Instructions
1. Lie on the back with the ball under the sacrum with the knees bent and both feet on the mat.
2. Flex the right hip and bend the right knee so it is at a 90-degree angle. Clasp both hands behind the right knee.

3. Inhale to initiate.
4. Exhale, extending the right knee above the body as much as feels comfortable.
5. Gently pull the right leg slightly toward the body until the hamstring lengthens.
6. Hold for 5 to 10 seconds, breathing normally.
7. Repeat on the other side.
8. Perform as needed on each side, completing the repetitions on one side of the body before switching sides.

Alignment Cues

- Move slowly and do not bounce or pulse.
- Keep the stretch comfortable, not painful.
- Always keep a slight soft bend in the knees when stretching the hamstrings.

SAFETY TIP Those with tight hamstrings may use a towel or band to gently pull the leg toward the body.

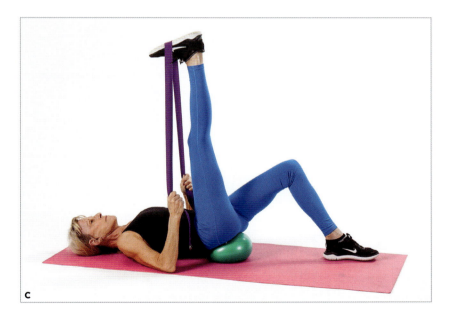
c

Upper Back and Chest Stretch

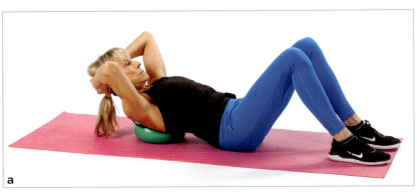

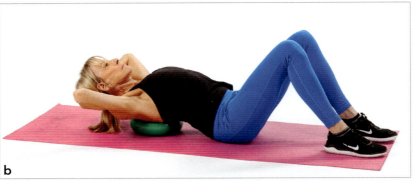

Benefits
Placing the ball between the shoulder blades allows for greater thoracic extension.

Instructions
1. Lie on the back on a mat with the ball between the shoulder blades, placing the hands behind the head to support the head and neck and keeping the elbows near the ears.
2. Inhale to initiate.
3. Exhale to gently extend the spine, keeping the head elevated and supported.
4. If there are no shoulder impingements, slightly abduct the elbows.
5. Hold for 5 to 10 seconds, breathing normally.
6. Return to the starting position.
7. Perform as many repetitions as needed.

Alignment Cues
- Move slowly and with intention.
- Always support the head.
- Only move until you feel a gentle stretch in the pectoralis.
- Keep the hips on the floor throughout the movement.

SAFETY TIP Place a rolled-up towel under the head for support. Please note that this stretch should not be performed by anyone with neck issues.

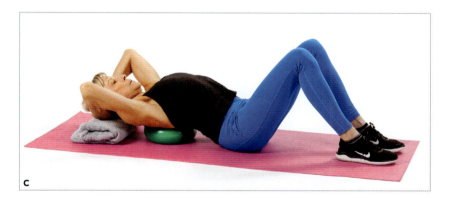

c

PART III

Workouts

CHAPTER 9

Create Workouts

The workouts in part III are designed to give you examples of a program using exercises chosen to meet a specific goal. A consistent core training program is not only essential to a fitness and wellness routine, but it will increase core strength, mobility, and stability in all other daily activities. You can choose a variety of exercises and stretches to fit client goals and diversify their workouts. Employing a wide selection of exercises is vital to preventing overuse injuries and boredom. These exercises can also complement other forms of training such as cardiovascular or resistance training to complete a well-rounded fitness plan.

Encourage clients to consult with a medical professional before starting an exercise program if they have any limitations, and remind them to be aware of how they feel as they move. Remember that not all exercises may be suitable for those with injuries or who are pregnant and that you may need to modify an exercise to make it appropriate. Because many of the exercises offer regressions and safety tips, you can find options that best suit each client.

Preparing for a Workout

The core workouts in part III require that the mind and body work together synergistically to create a stronger core, decrease pain, and improve functionality. In order to experience these benefits, a client must commit to truly feeling the exercise in their body. If any movement does not feel right or causes discomfort, an alternative should be given.

As you work with clients, it may be helpful to follow these guidelines:

- *Familiarize yourself with the purpose of each exercise.* Take time to get familiar with each exercise and how to cue it, especially if you are new to using a small ball in core training. Starting a new program requires the body and mind to adjust to new concepts of training, especially when using specific stimuli such as the small ball. It is one thing to simply perform the exercises, but as a trainer, you need to be able to convey the purpose of each exercise and demonstrate how to do it correctly. Practice the exercises so you can describe to your clients where they should feel an exercise and why.

- *Emphasize presence and control.* Executing an exercise involves consciously moving for a subconscious result. In other words, the exercises are designed to move the body authentically and without restraint. A client should never squeeze, tighten, or tuck the hips, placing the spine in a compromised position. Encourage them to concentrate on staying present and paying attention to the movement. Moving slowly and allowing the sensation of the movement to happen allows the body to respond naturally and functionally.

- *Remember to breathe.* Not only does the breath enhance the movement, but it calms the nervous system to allow the body to perform with greater ease and less tension. Breathing through the movement lets the core muscles that are responsible for respiration authentically engage. Breathing also improves blood circulation and oxygenation to the targeted muscles, thus increasing efficacy. It is not necessary to breathe so deeply that you lose rhythm; keep the breath natural, moving in through the nose and out through the mouth.

- *Be patient.* Those who are new to small ball core training will probably experience a bit of frustration because some exercises may feel counterintuitive. Traditional core exercises, such as abdominal crunches, cause a shortening of the anterior core, whereas the exercises in this book emphasize lengthening the muscles and fasciae against gravity. The muscles are still working, and sensations such as shaking while performing an exercise may occur until the muscles get stronger. The strength will come with consistent and dedicated practice.

- *Maintain alignment.* It is never necessary to push harder to achieve better results, and you should never encourage a client to move farther into a position than necessary. Remember that the old adage "no pain, no gain" can lead to injuries, especially to the back. Align the spine in the correct position before initiating an exercise to ensure the best outcome. Practitioners should familiarize themselves with the potential mistakes that clients make while executing the exercises and stretches. Improperly performing a stretch may not result in injury, but it can mean lesser or even no benefit for the targeted muscles, and practitioners can learn to predict those pitfalls before they happen.

Safety Tips

- Make sure that the ball is placed in the correct position for each exercise.
- Make sure that the exercise is at the appropriate fitness level.
- Make sure regressions or progressions for each exercise are adequate for different ability levels.
- Make sure to keep the spine neutral.
- Make sure to breathe normally.
- Make sure to move slowly to feel the exercise and its purpose.
- Make sure to work within the appropriate range of motion.
- Make sure to follow the cues correctly based on the exercise.

Warm-Up for All Levels

It is always important to move the body in preparation for any activity, whether core work or cardio. The warm-up stimulates the brain and prepares the body for work. Clients who are alert and physically prepared will be better able to focus on their movements and are less likely to be injured.

Breath Work

Perform as needed to feel how your breath activates the deep core muscles.

Holding the Ball
1. While standing, hold the ball in front of the body.
2. Inhale to initiate.
3. Exhale and press gently into the ball with the hands.
4. Perform 6 to 8 repetitions.

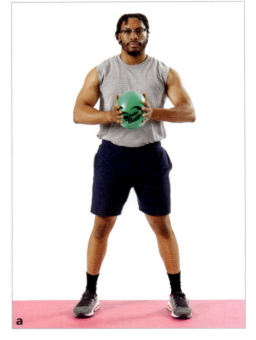

Standing With the Ball
1. Still standing, place the ball between the thighs just above the knees.
2. Inhale to initiate.
3. Exhale to engage the inner thighs, pressing against the ball and lifting through the pelvic floor.
4. While engaging the inner thighs, stay focused on activating the deep core muscles.
5. Hold for 5 to 10 seconds. Perform 6 to 8 repetitions.

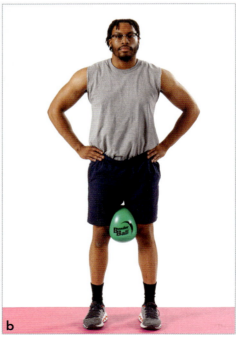

Squatting With the Ball

1. Keep the ball between the thighs.
2. Inhale to initiate and lower the hips into a shallow squat.
3. Exhale to return to standing as you press the thighs against the ball. Keep the inner thighs engaged to activate the deep core muscles.
4. Perform 6 to 8 repetitions.

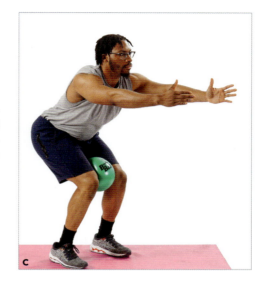

Dynamic Stretches

Perform as many repetitions as needed of each of the following movements.

Squat

1. Hold the ball in both hands in front of the chest with the feet hip-width apart.
2. Inhale to initiate the squat.
3. Exhale to return, straightening the knees and reaching both arms upward.
4. For a progression, place the ball in between the thighs.

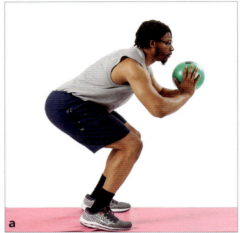
a

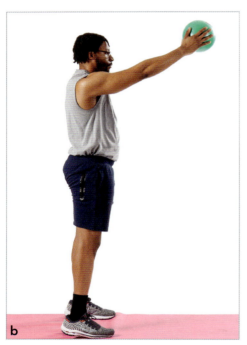
b

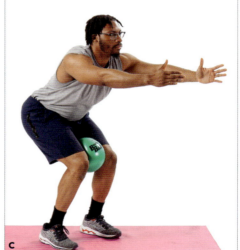
c

Lateral Bend

1. Holding the ball in both hands, lift the arms over the head.
2. Inhale to initiate.
3. Exhale to laterally flex.
4. Flex the torso from right to left, keeping the spine lengthened.

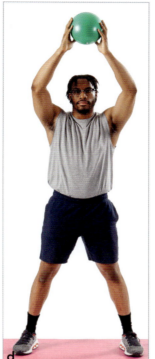
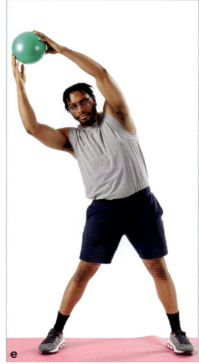

Spinal Rotation

1. Hold the ball in both hands in front of the chest.
2. Inhale to initiate.
3. Exhale and rotate the spine to the right and left.
4. At the same time, rotate the hips from right to left.

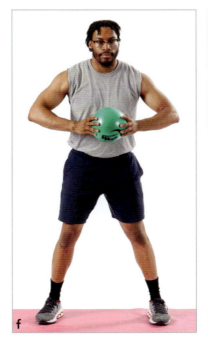
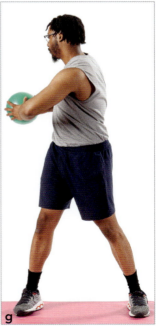

Core Essentials Workouts

Each of the following workouts offer challenge and a variety of exercises according to client fitness levels and abilities. Any of the exercises can be regressed or progressed as appropriate for individual client needs. The amount of time spent on each workout can also be adjusted based on number of repetitions performed and client goals.

Beginning Core Essentials

The client who is just starting a core program may not have innate body awareness and coordination; therefore, it is best to start at a slow pace and let the exercise sink in. The novice may not know whether they are doing an exercise correctly; it is up to you as the trainer to guide them. Like any other activity, there is a cognitive stage to learning core training. One does not pick up a golf club and immediately become an expert, but with time, practice, and coaching, one has a chance to become proficient.

This beginning core program, shown in table 9.1, is slightly shorter and less intense than the others and allows the client to focus on alignment and form prior to advancing. It is important to direct their focus to moving slowly and experiencing how the breath can enhance strength, balance, and functionality.

TABLE 9.1 Beginning Core Essentials

Exercise	Image	Cue	Page
Parallel Squat (Ball Between Thighs)		Keep a lengthened, neutral spine and the knees aligned with the toes.	26
Calf and Posterior Hip Lengthening		Keep a lengthened, neutral spine with the toes facing forward.	27

Exercise	Image	Cue	Page
Anterior Hip Lengthening		Keep a lengthened, neutral spine as you reach the arms overhead.	28
Squat With Lateral Flexion and Rotation		Keep the spine lengthened and the knees in a pain-free range.	32
Hip Flexion and Balance		Flex the hip only to 90 degrees and focus on the supporting hip.	42
Kneeling (Ball Between Thighs)		Engage the inner thighs to activate the deep core muscles.	61

(continued)

Table 9.1 Beginning Core Essentials *(continued)*

Exercise	Image	Cue	Page
Kneeling With Lateral Flexion (Ball Between Thighs)		Flex the spine only enough to feel the lateral core muscles engage.	62
Hands and Knees (Ball Under Hand)		Keep the spine neutral and engage the deep core muscles.	68
Hands and Knees With Glider Disc (Ball Between Thighs)		Engage the adductors to activate the deep core muscles.	73
Side-Lying Lateral Flexion (Ball Under Side)		Engage the lateral core muscles.	94
Side-Lying Hip Abduction (Ball Under Head)		Engage the lateral core muscles and hip abductors.	104
Seated Anterior Core Lengthening (Ball Behind Low Back)		Engage and lengthen the anterior core muscles.	116

Exercise	Image	Cue	Page
Seated Anterior and Lateral Core Rotation (Ball Behind Low Back)		Engage and lengthen the anterior and lateral core muscles.	122
Bridge (Ball Under Sacrum)		Engage and lengthen the anterior core muscles.	127
Bridge (Ball Between Knees)		Engage the deep core muscles.	128
Toe Taps (Ball Under Sacrum)		Engage the deep core muscles and focus on balance.	136
Thread the Needle		Lengthen and stretch the posterior core.	158
Supine Rotation		Lengthen and stretch the lateral core.	162

Intermediate Core Essentials

The intermediate core workout (table 9.2) adds challenge and takes more time to complete than the beginner workout. It is ideal for the client who is ready to explore new exercises. Just as some individuals may pick up golf more quickly than others, some clients may progress more efficiently through the exercises. Keep in mind that these exercises are designed to be safe for all participants.

TABLE 9.2 Intermediate Core Essentials

Exercise	Image	Cue	Page
Calf and Posterior Hip Lengthening		Lengthen the spine with the toes facing forward.	27
Anterior Hip Lengthening		Lengthen the spine and hip flexors.	28
Staggered Squat (Ball Between Thighs)		Lengthen the spine and engage the deep core muscles.	29

Create Workouts 187

Exercise	Image	Cue	Page
Squat With Lateral Flexion and Rotation		Lengthen the spine and keep the knees in alignment.	32
Curtsy Lunge With Glider Disc		Lengthen the spine and hinge with a neutral spine.	34
Hands and Knees With Hip Extension (Ball Under Hand)		Keep the spine neutral.	70
Plank (Ball Between Thighs)		Lift out of the shoulders with a neutral spine and engage the deep core muscles.	83
Plank With Rotation (Ball Between Thighs)		Lift out of the shoulders and rotate only until the lateral core is engaged.	86
Forearm Plank With Hip Rotation With Glider Disc (Ball Between Thighs)		Lift out of the shoulders and rotate the hips only until the lateral core is engaged.	89

(continued)

Table 9.2 Intermediate Core Essentials *(continued)*

Exercise	Image	Cue	Page
Side-Lying Hip Adduction (Ball Between Ankles)		Lift the hips slightly and focus on the lateral core.	98
Forearm Side Plank (Ball Between Thighs)		Engage the inner thighs to activate the deep core muscles.	100
Side-Lying Hip Abduction and Lateral Flexion (Ball Under Side)		Laterally flex and extend to engage the lateral core.	108
Seated Anterior Core Lengthening With Chair		Engage the anterior core and lift the arms within the appropriate range of motion.	118
Seated Anterior Core Lengthening With Glider Disc (Ball Behind Low Back)		Engage the anterior core and lift the arms and extend the hips within the appropriate range of motion.	120
Seated Anterior and Lateral Core Rotation With Glider Disc (Ball Behind Low Back)		Engage the anterior and lateral core and rotate within the appropriate range of motion.	124
Seated Anterior Core Lengthening (Ball Behind Mid Back)		Extend the spine only until the anterior core lengthens.	115

Create Workouts | 189

Exercise	Image	Cue	Page
Seated Anterior and Lateral Core Lengthening (Ball Behind Mid Back)		Lengthen the front of the body while laterally flexing.	126
Bridge (Ball Between Knees)		Lift to a neutral bridge and activate the adductors to engage the deep core muscles.	128
Bridge (Ball Under Foot)		Lift to a neutral bridge and focus on balance.	130
Bridge (Ball on Thighs)		Lift to a neutral bridge and add enough pressure on the ball to engage the deep core muscles.	132
Hip and Knee Extension (Ball Under Sacrum)		Lower the extended hip to 45 degrees.	138
Side-Lying Stretch		Place the ball in a supportive position to lengthen the side body and lift through the lateral core.	160
Supine Rotation		Place the ball under the knee for elevation.	162
Hip Flexor Stretch		Place the ball under one buttock at a time.	166

Advanced Core Essentials

The advanced core workout (table 9.3) is intended for those clients who have good control and body awareness and want to ramp up the challenge level of their core training. This client is more autonomous and has mastered movement and proficiency. Even with the more challenging core exercises, safety should not be compromised.

TABLE 9.3 Advanced Core Essentials

Exercise	Image	Cue	Page
Calf and Posterior Hip Lengthening		Lengthen the spine with the toes facing forward.	27
Anterior Hip Lengthening		Lengthen the spine and hip flexors.	28
Curtsy Lunge With Glider Disc		Lengthen the spine and hinge with a neutral spine.	34

Exercise	Image	Cue	Page
Lunge		Hinge with a neutral spine.	36
Squat to Balance		Lift from the supporting hip and lift through the core.	40
Balance (Ball Under Foot)		Lift through the supporting side and apply light pressure on the ball.	52
Hands and Knees With Hip Extension (Ball Under Knee)		Keep the spine neutral and lift out of the shoulders.	72
Plank With Hip Extension (Ball Between Thighs)		Keep the spine neutral and lift out of the shoulders. Engage the adductors to activate the deep core muscles.	84

(continued)

Table 9.3 Advanced Core Essentials *(continued)*

Exercise	Image	Cue	Page
Plank With Rotation (Ball Between Thighs)		Keep the spine neutral, lift out of the shoulders, and rotate only until the lateral core is engaged.	86
Forearm Plank With Hip Rotation With Glider Disc (Ball Between Thighs)		Engage the adductors and rotate the hips only until the lateral core is engaged.	89
Forearm Plank (Ball Between Hands)		Lift out of the shoulders and engage the deep core muscles.	90
Prone Spinal Extension (Ball Under Hands)		Lift only until the anterior body is lengthened and do not hyperextend the spine.	91
Side-Lying Lateral Flexion With Glider Disc (Ball Under Side)		Laterally flex only until the lateral core is engaged.	96
Side-Lying Hip Adduction (Ball Between Ankles)		Lift the hips only until the lateral core is engaged.	98
One-Handed Side Plank (Ball Between Thighs)		Lift out of the shoulders and engage the adductors until the deep core muscles are engaged.	102

Create Workouts 193

Exercise	Image	Cue	Page
Side-Lying Hip Abduction and Lateral Flexion With Glider Disc (Ball Under Side)		Laterally flex only until the lateral core is engaged and keep the thigh even with the hip.	110
Seated Anterior Core Lengthening (Ball Behind Low Back)		Lift the arms only until the anterior core is engaged.	116
Seated Anterior Core Lengthening With Glider Disc (Ball Behind Low Back)		Lift the arms only until the anterior core is engaged and keep the feet on the glider disc.	120
Seated Anterior and Lateral Core Rotation With Glider Disc (Ball Behind Low Back)		Lift the arms only until the anterior core is engaged and keep the feet on the glider disc.	124
Seated Anterior and Lateral Core Lengthening (Ball Behind Mid Back)		Move only until the anterior lateral core is engaged.	126
Hip Flexion (Ball on Thigh)		Keep the spine neutral and engage the deep core muscles.	140

(continued)

Table 9.3 Advanced Core Essentials *(continued)*

Exercise	Image	Cue	Page
Inner Thigh Stretch		Abduct the thighs only until a stretch is felt.	154
Hip Flexor Stretch		Place the ball under one buttock at a time.	166
Hamstring Stretch		Stretch the hamstring within a comfortable range of motion.	168

CHAPTER 10

Workouts for Better Posture and a Healthy Back

In this chapter you will be able to choose a variety of exercises and stretches that are specifically designed to address postural and back issues. Back pain is one of the leading causes of dysfunction and a poor quality of life, and many postural dysfunctions are a result of improper core training. Teaching a functionally safer approach to core training and strengthening the body's core in a multitude of positions and planes of motion using a small ball will help keep the back strong for life.

Before using these workouts, review the Preparing for a Workout section starting on page 176 in chapter 9. Keep in mind that if your client has a postural issue or low back pain, knowing the purpose of each exercise you choose is vital for success. Remember that not every exercise is appropriate for each student; modify and offer alternatives as needed to ensure safety and reduce the risk of injury.

Exercises for Everyday Function

We sometimes take for granted how vital it is that we have a strong core for daily functioning. In the workout program shown in table 10.1, exercises have been specifically chosen to help clients meet the demands of daily life, from gardening to working. You will see that many of the exercises are performed in a vertical position, which is most similar to our natural positioning throughout the day—sitting, reaching, walking, and more. You will find these exercises beneficial for all clients.

TABLE 10.1 Exercises for Everyday Function

Exercise	Image	Cue	Page
Parallel Squat (Ball Between Thighs)		Keep a lengthened, neutral spine and the knees aligned with the toes.	26
Calf and Posterior Hip Lengthening		Keep the spine neutral with the toes facing forward.	27
Anterior Hip Lengthening		Keep the spine neutral as you reach the arms above the shoulders.	28

Workouts for Better Posture and a Healthy Back

Exercise	Image	Cue	Page
Parallel Squat (Ball Between Hands)		Keep the spine lengthened and the knees in a pain-free range.	30
Squat With Lateral Flexion and Rotation		Keep the spine lengthened and the knees in a pain-free range.	32
Curtsy Lunge With Glider Disc		Keep the spine lengthened and hinge with a neutral spine.	34
Lunge		Keep the spine lengthened and hinge with a neutral spine.	36

(continued)

Table 10.1 Exercises for Everyday Function *(continued)*

Exercise	Image	Cue	Page
Squat to Balance		Keep the spine lengthened and the knees in a pain-free range.	40
Hip Flexion and Balance		Flex the hip only to 90 degrees and focus on the supporting hip.	42
Two-Handed Wall Press		Keep the spine lengthened and the hips wide for balance.	44
Balance (Ball Under Foot)		Keep the spine lengthened and apply light pressure to the ball.	52

Workouts for Better Posture and a Healthy Back

Exercise	Image	Cue	Page
Kneeling With Lateral Flexion (Ball Between Thighs)		Keep the spine lengthened and engage the adductors.	62
Kneeling With Rotation (Ball Between Thighs)		Lift and lengthen the spine, and only move the hips slightly from right to left and vice versa.	64
Forearm Plank (Ball Under Chest)		Lift out of the shoulders, keep the spine neutral, and engage the core.	81
Plank to Pike With Glider Disc (Ball Between Thighs)		Lift out of the shoulders, lift the hips, and engage the core.	88
Side-Lying Lateral Flexion (Ball Under Side)		Engage the lateral core muscles.	94
Side-Lying Lateral Flexion With Glider Disc (Ball Under Side)		Engage the lateral core muscles while sliding the hand.	96

(continued)

Table 10.1 Exercises for Everyday Function *(continued)*

Exercise	Image	Cue	Page
Seated Anterior Core Lengthening (Ball Behind Low Back)		Engage and lengthen the anterior core muscles.	116
Seated Anterior Core Lengthening With Chair		Engage and lengthen the anterior core muscles.	118
Seated Anterior Core Lengthening With Glider Disc (Ball Behind Low Back)		Engage and lengthen the anterior core muscles.	120
Seated Anterior and Lateral Core Rotation (Ball Behind Low Back)		Engage and lengthen the anterior and lateral core muscles.	122
Seated Anterior and Lateral Core Rotation With Glider Disc (Ball Behind Low Back)		Engage and lengthen the anterior and lateral core muscles.	124

Workouts for Better Posture and a Healthy Back

Exercise	Image	Cue	Page
Seated Anterior Core Lengthening (Ball Behind Mid Back)		Engage and lengthen the anterior core muscles.	115
Side Bend		Lengthen through the spine while laterally flexing.	148
Side Bend With Legs Crossed		Gently press into the hip for greater flexibility.	150
Posterior Cross Lunge		Lengthen through the spine and hinge forward to stretch the hip.	152

(continued)

Table 10.1 Exercises for Everyday Function *(continued)*

Exercise	Image	Cue	Page
Inner Thigh Stretch		Keep the spine lengthened and do not overstretch.	154
Hamstring Stretch		Keep the knees soft.	168

Exercises for Lordosis

The workout in table 10.2 is designed to address lordosis (a postural issue discussed in chapter 2). The exercises are specifically selected to strengthen the anterior core and glutes and deactivate the hip flexors, which are commonly overused in most core exercises. Placing the ball behind the low back is an essential tool in deactivating the hip flexors.

TABLE 10.2 Exercises for Lordosis

Exercise	Image	Cue	Page
Calf and Posterior Hip Lengthening		Lengthen the spine while hinging forward.	27

Workouts for Better Posture and a Healthy Back   **203**

Exercise	Image	Cue	Page
Anterior Hip Lengthening		Lengthen the spine as you reach the arms above the shoulders (do not arch the back).	28
Curtsy Lunge With Glider Disc		Lengthen the spine and hinge with a neutral spine.	34
Lunge		Lengthen the spine to engage the glutes.	36
Lunge With Glider Disc		Lengthen the spine to engage the glutes.	38

(continued)

Table 10.2 Exercises for Lordosis *(continued)*

Exercise	Image	Cue	Page
Back Press to Wall		Lengthen the anterior core.	48
Hands and Knees With Glider Disc (Ball Between Thighs)		Keep the spine neutral.	73
Plank to Pike With Glider Disc (Ball Between Thighs)		Keep the spine neutral.	88
Side-Lying Lateral Flexion (Ball Under Side)		Stay lengthened and do not collapse the ribs into the ball.	94
Side-Lying Hip Abduction (Ball Under Head)		Stay lengthened in the side body and do not lift the hip too high.	104
Seated Anterior Core Lengthening (Ball Behind Low Back)		Lengthen the anterior core and disengage the hip flexors.	116

Workouts for Better Posture and a Healthy Back

Exercise	Image	Cue	Page
Seated Anterior Core Lengthening With Chair		Lengthen the anterior core and disengage the hip flexors.	118
Seated Anterior Core Lengthening With Glider Disc (Ball Behind Low Back)		Use the anterior core when flexing and extending the hip instead of the hip flexors.	120
Seated Anterior and Lateral Core Rotation (Ball Behind Low Back)		Lengthen the anterior core and lift when rotating the lateral core.	122
Seated Anterior and Lateral Core Rotation With Glider Disc (Ball Behind Low Back)		Lengthen the anterior core and lift when rotating the lateral core.	124
Seated Anterior Core Lengthening (Ball Behind Mid Back)		Lengthen the anterior core.	115
Bridge (Ball Under Sacrum)		Lengthen the anterior core while keeping the hips supported.	127

(continued)

Table 10.2 Exercises for Lordosis *(continued)*

Exercise	Image	Cue	Page
Bridge (Ball Between Knees)		Lengthen the anterior core and engage the adductors.	128
Side Bend		Lengthen through the spine while laterally flexing.	148
Posterior Cross Lunge		Lengthen through the spine and hinge forward to engage the glutes.	152
Inner Thigh Stretch		Make sure not to overstretch.	154

Workouts for Better Posture and a Healthy Back

Exercise	Image	Cue	Page
Supine Rotation		Rotate only far enough to feel a stretch.	162
Hip Flexor Stretch		Lengthen the desired side by deep breathing.	166
Hamstring Stretch		Make sure not to overstretch.	168

Exercises for Kyphosis

The workout in table 10.3 is designed to address kyphosis (a postural issue discussed in chapter 2). The exercises are selected to promote better flexibility and mobility of the thoracic spine, particularly with a forward head position. Supporting the low back with the ball also promotes hamstring lengthening.

TABLE 10.3 Exercises for Kyphosis

Exercise	Image	Cue	Page
Calf and Posterior Hip Lengthening		Lengthen the spine while hinging forward.	27

(continued)

Table 10.3 Exercises for Kyphosis *(continued)*

Exercise	Image	Cue	Page
Anterior Hip Lengthening		Lengthen the spine and only reach the arms as far above the shoulders as comfortable.	28
Staggered Squat (Ball Between Thighs)		Lengthen the spine and keep more weight in the posterior hip.	29
Squat With Lateral Flexion and Rotation		Lengthen and lift the torso while laterally flexing and rotating.	32
Curtsy Lunge With Glider Disc		Lengthen the spine and hinge only until the lateral core is engaged.	34

Workouts for Better Posture and a Healthy Back **209**

Exercise	Image	Cue	Page
One-Handed Wall Press		Lengthen the spine, keep the feet wider than the hips for balance, and only apply slight pressure to the ball.	46
Back Press to Wall		Lengthen the spine, keep the feet wider than the hips, and press the thoracic spine into the ball.	48
Back Press to Wall With Rotation		Lengthen and rotate the spine with the feet wider than the hips.	49
Balance (Ball Outside Knee)		Lift through and engage the supporting side of the body.	56

(continued)

Table 10.3 Exercises for Kyphosis *(continued)*

Exercise	Image	Cue	Page
Kneeling With Lateral Flexion (Ball Between Thighs)		Lift through the torso while laterally flexing.	62
Kneeling With Rotation (Ball Between Thighs)		Lift through the torso while rotating.	64
Forearm Plank (Ball Under Chest)		Lift out of the shoulders and keep the spine neutral.	81
Side-Lying Lateral Flexion With Glider Disc (Ball Under Side)		Lengthen and engage the lateral core when laterally flexing and extending the spine.	96
Seated Anterior Core Lengthening (Ball Behind Low Back)		Lengthen the anterior core.	116

Workouts for Better Posture and a Healthy Back 211

Exercise	Image	Cue	Page
Seated Anterior Core Lengthening With Chair		Lengthen the anterior core.	118
Seated Anterior and Lateral Core Rotation (Ball Behind Low Back)		Lengthen the anterior and lateral core while rotating.	122
Seated Anterior Core Lengthening (Ball Behind Mid Back)		Extend the spine only far enough to lengthen the anterior core.	115
Side Bend		Lift and lengthen through the lateral core.	148

(continued)

Table 10.3 **Exercises for Kyphosis** *(continued)*

Exercise	Image	Cue	Page
Thread the Needle		Rotate only until a gentle stretch is felt.	158
Pectoralis Stretch		Stretch only as far as comfortable.	159
Supine Rotation		Stretch only as far as comfortable.	162
Hamstring Stretch		Make sure not to overstretch.	168
Upper Back and Chest Stretch		Make sure not to overstretch.	170

Exercises for a Healthy Back

In the workout in table 10.4, exercises have been specifically chosen that use the ball to protect the low back at all times. When the hip flexors are disengaged, the anterior core has a better opportunity to work. In each of these exercises, encourage the client to move only to the point where the core is engaged, without causing any discomfort in the back.

Note that for the purposes of this book, we offer specific exercises and stretches that promote a healthy back rather than rehabilitation. If any of your clients experience back issues or chronic pain, suggest that they seek the help of a medical professional for guidance.

> ### Safety Tips
>
> These exercises are intended to help decrease back discomfort and increase core strength. Although specific exercises have been suggested, each client is different. It is helpful to remember the following safety tips:
>
> - Never push to the point of discomfort or pain.
> - Do not recommend an exercise that is inappropriate for a client's needs.
> - Move within the appropriate range of motion.
> - Only choose the exercises that feel good to the back.
> - Focus on breathing.
> - Always have the ball in the correct location to protect the back.

TABLE 10.4 Exercises for a Healthy Back

Exercise	Image	Cue	Page
Calf and Posterior Hip Lengthening		Lengthen the spine while hinging forward.	27
Anterior Hip Lengthening		Lengthen the spine but do not arch the back.	28

(continued)

Table 10.4 Exercises for a Healthy Back *(continued)*

Exercise	Image	Cue	Page
Two-Handed Wall Press		Keep the feet wider than the hips and gently press into the ball.	44
Back Press to Wall		Keep the feet wider than the hips for balance.	48
Back Press to Wall With Rotation		Keep the feet wider than the hips for balance and rotate slowly.	49
Kneeling With Lateral Flexion (Ball Between Thighs)		Lift the torso off the ribs and lengthen the spine.	62

Workouts for Better Posture and a Healthy Back 215

Exercise	Image	Cue	Page
Kneeling With Rotation (Ball Between Thighs)		Lift and lengthen the spine, and only move the hips slightly from right to left and vice versa.	64
Seated Anterior Core Lengthening (Ball Behind Low Back)		Lengthen the anterior core.	116
Seated Anterior Core Lengthening With Chair		Lengthen the anterior core.	118
Seated Anterior and Lateral Core Rotation (Ball Behind Low Back)		Lengthen the anterior and lateral core and move slowly into rotation.	122
Seated Anterior Core Lengthening (Ball Behind Mid Back)		Lengthen the anterior core.	115
Bridge (Ball Under Sacrum)		Lengthen the anterior core while keeping the back supported.	127

(continued)

Table 10.4 Exercises for a Healthy Back *(continued)*

Exercise	Image	Cue	Page
Bridge (Ball Between Knees)		Lengthen the anterior core and engage the adductors.	128
Side Bend		Lengthen through the spine while laterally flexing.	148
Inner Thigh Stretch		Stretch the inner thighs only as far as needed.	154
Side-Lying Stretch		Make sure the ball is supporting the side body.	160
Supine Rotation		Place the ball under the knee for elevation.	162
Hip Flexor Stretch		Place only part of the ball under the buttock for elevation and do not hyperextend the spine.	166

Exercise	Image	Cue	Page
Hamstring Stretch		Make sure the ball is in a comfortable position to allow the hamstrings to stretch.	168

Restorative Stretches

The ball provides support for many clients to enjoy benefits of stretching that they may otherwise be unable to achieve. Cue clients to never overstretch, nor to stretch to the point of pain or discomfort. They should take deep breaths and gently move or hold for about 10 seconds to allow the body to relax. The stretches are designed to be included in all workout and fitness formats, and there are varying positions to choose from based on your clients' needs and activities.

These stretches are held, unlike those in a warm-up, which are more active. Even though the movements may look similar, the intention and purpose is different. The stretches in table 10.5 are designed to promote a healthier back and better posture and to relax and restore the body.

TABLE 10.5 Restorative Stretches

Exercise	Image	Cue	Page
Side Bend With Legs Crossed		Lengthen through the spine while laterally flexing.	150

(continued)

Table 10.5 Restorative Stretches *(continued)*

Exercise	Image	Cue	Page
Thread the Needle		Rotate only until a stretch is felt.	158
Pectoralis Stretch		Make sure to gently rest the arm on the ball.	159
Side-Lying Stretch		Lengthen the side body while relaxing on the ball.	160
Supine Rotation		Keep the knees elevated and relax into the lower back.	162
Butterfly Stretch		Allow the hips to open only as far as is comfortable.	164
Hip Flexor Stretch		Elevate the hip only until the stretch is felt in the hip flexor.	166
Hamstring Stretch		Make sure the ball is in a comfortable position to allow the hamstrings to stretch.	168
Upper Back and Chest Stretch		Make sure not to hyperextend the neck.	170

CHAPTER 11

Core Workouts for Rotational Sports

Rotational sports such as pickleball, tennis, and golf are a popular way to enjoy physical activity. These sports require you to move with momentum in all three planes of motion, which affects the entire body's core function. Many athletes know the importance of a well-balanced core routine to improve their game. However, if one does not train correctly, speed and agility can actually be inhibited, and injuries can occur.

When a sport is predominantly performed with one side of the body, it creates imbalances, which, if not addressed, will eventually cause injuries and dysfunctions as well. For example, the repetitive motion of swinging a golf club can cause shortening on one side of the body. Tennis and pickleball require much more rotation in the core, and because most people swing the racket more on one side of the body than the other, it is important to train the muscles throughout the core to encourage balance. Specific athletic core exercises will therefore not only strengthen the body but also create symmetry and better performance.

The exercises and stretches recommended in this chapter are a good balance of integrated training for these rotational sports, promoting better functionality, strength, flexibility, and overall performance. The exercises in each workout have been chosen for the intensity and demand of the sport.

Exercises for Pickleball

Pickleball is the fastest growing rotational sport in the country. It is a low-impact, easy-to-learn paddle sport that appeals to people of all ages and skill levels. This sport can be played either singles or doubles, indoors or outdoors, and takes place on a badminton court using a perforated plastic baseball and small paddles. Pickleball players do not have to move around as much as tennis players, so this sport can still be enjoyed by the active aging or by people with some physical limitations.

Although it is the least strenuous of the rotational sports, clients will benefit from training the core muscles used in the sport. The exercises in table 11.1 will help clients have a better experience in the game.

TABLE 11.1 Exercises for Pickleball

Exercise	Image	Cue	Page
Calf and Posterior Hip Lengthening		Hinge forward and keep the spine neutral.	27
Staggered Squat (Ball Between Thighs)		Hinge from the hips and keep the spine neutral.	29
Squat With Lateral Flexion and Rotation		Keep the spine lengthened.	32
Curtsy Lunge With Glider Disc		Keep the spine lengthened and hinge from the hips.	34

Core Workouts for Rotational Sports   221

Exercise	Image	Cue	Page
Kneeling With Lateral Flexion (Ball Between Thighs)		Engage the inner thighs while laterally flexing.	62
Hands and Knees With Hip Mobility With Glider Disc (Ball Between Thighs)		Lift out of the shoulders and slightly rotate the hips.	74
Plank With Rotation (Ball Between Thighs)		Keep the spine neutral when rotating.	86
Side-Lying Lateral Flexion (Ball Under Side)		Support the head with the hand.	94
Side-Lying Hip Abduction (Ball Under Head)		Abduct the thigh only until even with the hip.	104
Seated Anterior Core Lengthening (Ball Behind Low Back)		Lengthen the anterior core.	116

(continued)

Table 11.1 Exercises for Pickleball *(continued)*

Exercise	Image	Cue	Page
Seated Anterior and Lateral Core Rotation (Ball Behind Low Back)		Lengthen the anterior and lateral core.	122
Bridge (Ball Under Sacrum)		Lengthen the anterior core.	127
Bridge (Ball Between Knees)		Lengthen the anterior core and engage the adductors.	128
Toe Taps (Ball Under Sacrum)		Engage the core for balance.	136
Side Bend With Legs Crossed		Lengthen through the spine while laterally flexing.	150
Supine Rotation		Place the ball under the knee for elevation.	162
Hip Flexor Stretch		Position only a portion of the ball under the buttock for elevation.	166

Core Workouts for Rotational Sports 223

Exercises for Tennis

Tennis is a racket sport appropriate for all ages and skill levels. The sport can be played either singles or doubles on an indoor or outdoor court. Tennis requires more energy than pickleball, along with a stronger core and faster reaction time. It requires a lot of lateral and rotational movement while moving quickly to hit the ball with force; the most common sites of pain and injury among tennis players are centered in the low back and shoulders. The exercises in this workout, shown in table 11.2, were specifically chosen to help strengthen the core for this higher demand on the body.

TABLE 11.2 Exercises for Tennis

Exercise	Image	Cue	Page
Calf and Posterior Hip Lengthening		Keep the spine lengthened and the heel on the ground.	27
Anterior Hip Lengthening		Keep the spine lengthened.	28
Curtsy Lunge With Glider Disc		Keep the spine lengthened while hinging forward.	34

(continued)

Table 11.2 Exercises for Tennis *(continued)*

Exercise	Image	Cue	Page
Hands and Knees (Ball Under Hand)		Keep the core engaged and the spine neutral, with the supporting hand directly under the shoulder.	68
Hands and Knees With Hip Extension (Ball Under Hand)		Keep the core engaged and the spine neutral, with the supporting hand directly under the shoulder.	70
Forearm Plank (Ball Under Chest)		Keep the core engaged and the spine neutral; float the chest off of the ball.	81
Side-Lying Lateral Flexion (Ball Under Side)		Lengthen through the spine, creating space between the ribs and hip.	94
Side-Lying Lateral Flexion With Glider Disc (Ball Under Side)		Lengthen through the spine, creating space between the ribs and hip while sliding the hand.	96
Forearm Side Plank (Ball Between Thighs)		Keep the spine neutral and engage the adductors.	100
Seated Anterior Core Lengthening (Ball Behind Low Back)		Keep the spine lengthened while gazing upward.	116
Seated Anterior Core Lengthening With Glider Disc (Ball Behind Low Back)		Keep the spine lengthened while extending and flexing the hips and knees.	120

Core Workouts for Rotational Sports

Exercise	Image	Cue	Page
Seated Anterior and Lateral Core Rotation (Ball Behind Low Back)		Keep the spine lengthened while rotating.	122
Bridge (Ball on Thighs)		Lengthen the front of the body but do not engage the glutes.	132
Side Bend		Lengthen the spine and lift through the hips.	148
Side Bend With Legs Crossed		Lengthen through the hips, focusing on the lateral hip.	150

(continued)

Table 11.2 Exercises for Tennis *(continued)*

Exercise	Image	Cue	Page
Inner Thigh Stretch		Abduct the thighs only until a mild stretch is felt.	154
Thread the Needle		Cross the arm under the chest only until a mild stretch is felt in the shoulder.	158
Supine Rotation		Place the ball under the knee for elevation.	162
Hip Flexor Stretch		Position only a portion of the ball under the buttock for elevation and relax into the stretch.	166

Exercises for Golf

Golf is a popular sport for people of all ages and skill levels and can be done both individually or as part of a team. It requires coordination and precision as well as rotational speed. The main issue experienced by golfers is chronic low back pain. The exercises chosen for the workout in table 11.3 will help decrease the risk of injuries to the low back and knees. With correct core training, clients can enjoy this game pain free and with full function.

Core Workouts for Rotational Sports

TABLE 11.3 Exercises for Golf

Exercise	Image	Cue	Page
Anterior Hip Lengthening		Lengthen the spine.	28
Squat With Lateral Flexion and Rotation		Lengthen the spine while laterally flexing.	32
Squat to Balance		Focus on the stabilizing side of the body.	40
Balance (Ball Under Foot)		Focus on the stabilizing side of the body.	52

(continued)

Table 11.3 Exercises for Golf *(continued)*

Exercise	Image	Cue	Page
Balance (Ball Inside Knee)		Focus on the stabilizing side of the body.	54
Hands and Knees With Hip Extension (Ball Under Hand)		Lift out of the shoulders and keep the spine lengthened.	70
Hands and Knees With Hip Mobility With Glider Disc (Ball Between Thighs)		Keep the spine neutral and only move the hips slightly to engage the lateral core.	74
Side-Lying Lateral Flexion With Glider Disc (Ball Under Side)		Lift out of the shoulder and keep the spine long and neutral.	96
Side-Lying Hip Abduction and Lateral Flexion With Glider Disc (Ball Under Side)		Lift the thigh only to hip height.	110
Seated Anterior Core Lengthening (Ball Behind Low Back)		Lengthen the anterior core.	116

Core Workouts for Rotational Sports 229

Exercise	Image	Cue	Page
Seated Anterior and Lateral Core Rotation (Ball Behind Low Back)		Lengthen the anterior and lateral core.	122
Seated Anterior and Lateral Core Rotation With Glider Disc (Ball Behind Low Back)		Lengthen the anterior and lateral core and do not overutilize the hip flexors.	124
Bridge With Hip Flexion (Ball on Thigh)		Lengthen the anterior core and do not engage the glutes.	134
Toe Taps (Ball Under Sacrum)		Stabilize the body.	136
Side Bend		Lift and lengthen the spine when laterally flexing.	148

(continued)

Table 11.3 Exercises for Golf *(continued)*

Exercise	Image	Cue	Page
Side Bend With Legs Crossed		Lift and lengthen the spine when laterally flexing, holding the ball in the hands over the head.	150
Posterior Cross Lunge		Lengthen the spine when hinging forward.	152
Supine Rotation		Rotate only until a stretch is felt in the low back.	162
Hip Flexor Stretch		Position only a portion of the ball under the buttock and lengthen the hip flexor.	166
Upper Back and Chest Stretch		Make sure not to hyperextend the spine.	170

References

Chapter 1
Petrofsky, Jerrold S., Jennifer Batt, Nicceta Davis, Everett Lohman, Michael Laymon, Gerson E. De Leon, Heidi Roark, et al. 2007. "Core Muscle Activity During Exercise on a Mini Stability Ball Compared With Abdominal Crunches on the Floor and on a Swiss Ball." *Journal of Applied Research* 7, no. 3: 255-272. http://jarcet.com/articles/Vol7Iss3/PetrofskyVol7No3.pdf.

Chapter 2
Julia, Nina. 2023. "Chronic Back Pain Statistics in the US." Last modified January 11, 2024. https://cfah.org/back-pain-statistics/.

McGill, Stuart. 2002. *Low Back Disorders.* Champaign, IL: Human Kinetics.

About the Author

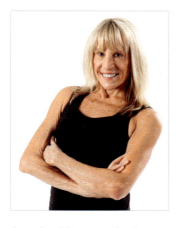

Leslee Bender, ACSM, NASM, FAFS, FAI, NPCP, is a 40-year veteran in the fitness industry and recipient of the 2020 IDEA Personal Trainer of the Year award. She is the coauthor of *I Am Ageless Now*, the owner of Ageless Now Academy, and the creator of the Bender Method of training, using the Bender Ball™.

Bender has presented worldwide and has appeared on national television. She has filmed video content for many companies, including Savvier, IDEA, Reebok, SCW, Ageless Academy, and more. The creator of Barre Above Pilates training and cocreator of Barre Above through Savvier Fitness, she has certified and trained thousands of fitness professionals internationally.

Bender is the programming director at Sports West Athletic Club in Reno, Nevada, where she trains all levels of students, specializing in pre- and postrehabilitative modalities. When in Florida, she works with professional athletes who compete in sports that emphasize rotational core movement, such as tennis and golf. She has a passion and love for the fitness industry and continues to grow and evolve her craft.

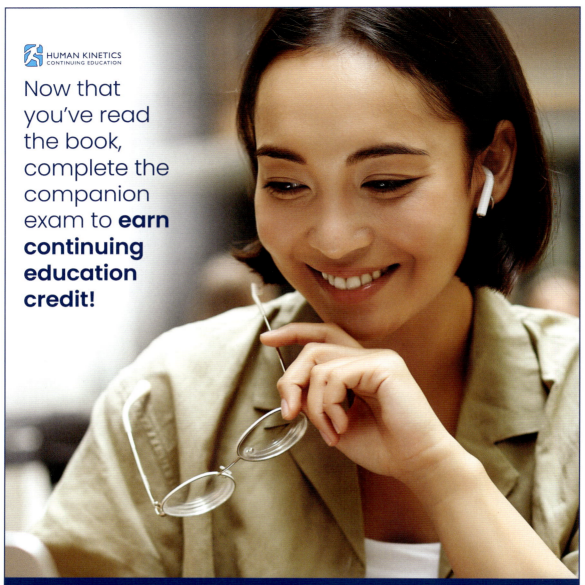